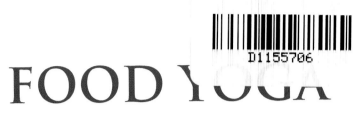

FOOD YOGA

Nourishing Body, Mind & Soul

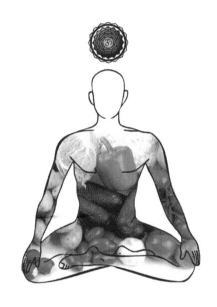

PAUL RODNEY TURNER
The Food Yogi

To my param guru, who taught me:
Spiritual evolution begins with the tongue

Table of Contents

THE SONG OF THE FOOD YOGI   9
ACKNOWLEDGEMENTS   11
FOREWORD   15
INTRODUCTION   17
FOOD YOGA   25
FOOD AND SCIENCE   29
    Food is Energy 29
    Quantum Physics 30
    Thoughts and Emotions are Energy 33
    Other Worlds 36
    Electromagnetic Spectrum 37
    Dark Energy 38
    The Superior Senses of Animals 39
    American Indians 43
    The Personification of Nature 46
    Intelligent Design 46
    Animism 49

WATER   51
    How Much Water Should I Drink? 53
    Food Yogi Rehydration Method 55
    Sacred Waters 57
    Energy Associations 60
    Water Memory 61
    Therapeutic Waters 62
    Water is a Conduit of Intention 62
    "I am the Taste of Water" 64
    First Steps in God Realization 66

WE ARE LOVED   69
    Nature Meditations 69
    Sacred Geometry of Whole Foods 71
    EARTH 75
    WATER 76
    FIRE 80
    AIR 81
    ETHER 81
    Sun Worship 83

FOOD POLITICS   89
    Is Your Food Safe? 89
    The Business of GMO 90
    The Power of the Plate 92
    The Dirty Dozen 93
    Commercial Milk 97

The CSA System 101
Grow Your Own Food 102
We Always Have a Choice 103
The Danger of Organic Foods 105
Veganic Agriculture 106
Biodynamic Agriculture 107
Food Laws... 108
Monsanto's Bait and Switch 110
Health Comes from Harmony...................................... 111

OUR TRUE NATURE   115
Solid Matter is an Illusion 115
Who Are We? 117
Spirits in a Material World 120
Yin Yang... 122

LIFE FORCES   125
Qi.. 125
The Electrical Body 126
Vital Energy 127
Prana.. 128
Breatharianism.. 132
Sun Gazing... 133

YOGA   139
Enlightened Karma Yoga... 143
A Yogi is Regulated 145
Laughter Yoga.. 146
Ecstatic Modifier... 147

YOGA AND AHIMSA   149
Yama and Niyama.. 152
The Yamas and Meat Eating.. 153

THE TONGUE   157
The Most Voracious of All the Senses 157
The Higher Taste.. 162
Lessons from the Ayurveda... 163
The Five Great Elements 164
The Three Doshas 164
The Six Tastes 166
Your Personal Constitution 168

THE POWER OF WORDS   171
Pure Sound 173
Gratitude.. 177

LIVING IN THE MOMENT   181
The Intention Experiment 182

Unique and Divine 184

THE GIFT OF FOOD   187

Food as a Medium of LOVE 187
You Have a Choice 188
Food Unites 189
How does Food Carry Intention? 190
Thanksgiving – a Day to Honor All Life 192
Compassion for Animals 197
The Karma connection 199

GOING BEYOND DIET   201

A Plant-Based Diet Is Not Enough 202
Mother's Love 203
The Seven Mothers 206
Food is a gift from MOTHER Earth 207
Offering Food Back to the Creators 207

THE FOOD YOGI DIET   209

Ahimsa 209
McVeggies 210
Eating the Way Nature Intended 211
The power of prasadam 213
How a dog achieved liberation 214
Prasadam can change the heart 215
Prisoners don't want to leave 217
Sraddha Ceremony 218

EVERYTHING WE DO   223

How do I become a Prasadarian? 225
How to Purify Your Meal 235
The Final Stage - The Offering 236

FOOD OFFERING MEDITATION   237

The Meaning of the Meditation 238

AFTER THE OFFERING   241

Sacred Eating 241
Conscious Eating Exercise 241
A Healthy Eating Regimen 249

INDIA'S VEDIC CULTURE OF HOSPITALITY   253

No One Should Go Hungry 253
The Meaning of Hospitality 254
The Story of King Rantideva 255

FOOD FOR LIFE   259

Mission 260
Aims and Objectives 260
"Uniting the World Through Pure Food" 261

Spiritual Equality 262
Universal Respect for All.. 264
Food for Life Projects 265
Emergency Food Relief 267
Children and Education... 269
Volunteer Diary 271
Testimonials 273

SACRED FOODS   277
FOOD YOGI SMOOTHIES   299
LIQUID MEALS 299
FRESH POWER JUICES 304
REFRESHERS 306

FERMENTED FOODS   309
CONCLUDING WORDS   315
APPENDIX   317
HOLY FOOD IN THE JUDEO-CHRISTIAN TRADITION   319
OFFERING FOOD IN BUDDHIST TRADITIONS   323
MERCY AND CHARITY IN THE ISLAMIC TRADITION   327
EATING AND CHARITY IN THE JEWISH TRADITION   331
SAINT FRANCIS OF ASSISI   335
ABOUT THE AUTHOR   339
RESOURCES   343
BIBLIOGRAPHY   345
START YOUR OWN PROJECT   347
For more information 348

The Song of the Food Yogi

As the soft moist grass folds beneath my feet,
I contemplate my good fortune and beg not to repeat,
The failures of the past in a journey so long,
There's just too much to tell in this very short song.
Holding my hands high, I reach for the sky,
personal liberation — I will not be denied,
By acting in ways that are averse to the course,
of the powerful waves — of that Illusory force.
I am far from perfect — and yet I feel so blessed,
by the saints that walked before me with egos undressed.
They now illuminate my path and guide my sorry plight,
in a world so overtaken by the fear of night.
Getting strength and vitality from the sun, water and air,
I embrace the divine love of the elemental fair,
as they nourish the teachings of the FOOD YOGA path,
and lead one and all to the Lord Jagannath.
The "Lord of the Universe," manifest within —
every atom of life and every tube-torus spin,
There is nowhere in our existence that God cannot be seen,
and that is essentially what FOOD YOGA means.
So honor your SELF — by honoring that Lord,
See thy presence manifest — in total accord,
with the degree of your love and openness of your heart,
And that my dear friend is where spirituality starts.
So engage your tongue properly — in respectable ways,
Don't chatter, offend — or eat horrible things today,
Purify the vibration — and the taste on your buds,
and experience the divine presence manifest from the mud —
Of a mischievous mind — submerged for far too long,
in matters of ignorance and sad love songs,
Realize your potential — beginning with your tongue,
and open your heart to the love of the divine ONE.

- The Food Yogi

Acknowledgements

My journey with this book began nearly 30 years ago when I was a monk helping other monks prepare meals for the needy in Australia. At that time, I watched in awe as head chef Garuda danced and sang around the kitchen while preparing a feast of vegetable curries, spicy rice, dhal, chutney, deep fried breads, semolina pudding, custard, cake and a refreshing drink. It was magic to behold. Here was a man, cooking for 200 people and just loving every minute of it. His infectious smile uplifted every one of us. Monk Garuda became my first culinary guru.

Soon after I was introduced to his teacher, Kurma Das, heralded as Australia's "Vegetarian Guru," who has kindly written the foreword to this book. Kurma has perfected the art and science of cooking for Krishna and has gone on to become a world-renowned chef and author of many amazing vegetarian cookbooks.

About a year later, I was introduced to Bhutanath, one of the all time great cooks in the Krishna movement. He was so talented, that the great grandson of Henry Ford, Alfred Ford, asked him to cater for his multi-million dollar wedding at the Bhaktivedanta Ashram in Colo River, Australia. I was one of "Bhuti's" kitchen staff. Years later when I became the head chef at the North Sydney Krishna temple, the award-winning chef and cookbook author Yamuna Devi became my constant source of inspiration. All these great souls were powerful influences in my early life and my food yoga journey.

In preparing this book, I must say that it could not have happened without the grace and inspiration of my two spiritual teachers, Srila Prabhupada[1] who taught me

---

[1] A Gaudiya Vaisnava teacher and the founder-acharya of the International Society for Krishna Consciousness.

everything I know about spiritual hospitality and food yoga, and Mukunda Goswami who clarified many of those teachings and inspired me to dedicate my life to the charity Food for Life Global (www.ffl.org) and the food yoga path.

There were many people that came into my life or my thoughts as this book was being revealed to me, first of which is my old friend Mahasringha ("Maha") whose compassion and unwavering determination to serve every one he meets blessed food, despite his own challenging circumstances, is just astonishing to witness. In many ways, he is the personification of what it means to be a food yogi.

The basis of this book came from notes of presentations I made at numerous vegetarian conferences around the world. Initially, the talks were called, "How to spiritualize your food," or "Spiritual Vegetarianism". During those early years, my close friends, Sandeep and Amrita Mody, Marilee Ash and Judy Campbell, encouraged my efforts and offered many valuable suggestions.

The initial manuscript began in New York during a low period in my life. It was a time of soul searching and rediscovering my core. Writing the book turned out to be therapy for my soul. I spent many all-night sessions at the famous 24-hour *Yaffa Café* in Manhattan, sipping rose petal tea and writing, sometimes not leaving the café until 9am to get an organic fruit smoothie from *Liquiteria* on 11th St.

As the book began to take shape, I asked for the opinions and suggestions of other close friends, including Gina Silvestri, the "Raw Food Muse". Her insight and encouragement were incredible. Maribeth Abrams of the North American Vegetarian Society also offered wonderful suggestions and critiques, and so too did vegan celebrity and award-winning author, Victoria Moran. My health coach, Melissa Klein of *Sun Compass Wellness* did an initial proofreading and offered invaluable feedback.

Nancy Adams of *Adams Communications* did a tremendous job in reorganizing the original structure of the book, while by my dear friend Gopali Nissen helped with proofreading. After many "incarnations" the final version was looked over by the brilliant Carol D'Costa of *Em and En Wordcraft*.

I am deeply grateful to all these wonderful people.

Finally, I thank all those that crossed my path on the food yoga journey and who directly or indirectly encouraged me in my service to Food for Life Global and my humble efforts to share this message to the world.

FOREWORD

It is an honor to have been asked to write a small foreword to this fascinating book. I have personally known Priyavrata for nearly 30 years. We have shared a common yoga path, and from time to time, we have found ourselves cooking together in kitchens around the world.

We both became inspired and empowered by the same teachings of the founder of ISKCON, Srila Prabhupada. From him we learned the art and science of Food Yoga. As explained in this book, one of the main elements of this yoga is the preparation of sacred foods. For thousands of years, kitchen yogis in temples throughout India have practiced the divine art and science of preparing wonderful and diverse vegetarian food saturated with love and devotion. Cooking thus becomes yoga.

The Sanskrit word yoga carries the meaning of 'connection', specifically the connection between the individual soul and the Supreme Soul. This connection has now been broken, and yoga is the means for re-establishing it.

The techniques for re-establishing the connection are intimate and personal. If we love someone, we want to do things for them, and a very common thing that people do for people they love is to cook for them.

Kitchen yogis around the world prepare offerings in this same spirit of love. This love is manifested at every stage of the cooking process – from growing or purchasing the ingredients to the final offering of the sacred meal to the object of one's devotion. Such a spiritualized diet is thus spiritually elevating.

If something is good for you spiritually, it is generally also good for you materially. Medical studies have shown that vegetarians tend to suffer less than others from various heart diseases and cancers. As far as the planet is concerned, the meat industry is one of the most wasteful of natural resources and the most destructive of the environment. A spiritual vegetarian diet is good not only for your soul but also for your body and our planet.

From this book you will learn how to achieve optimum health by practicing the Food Yogi diet and lifestyle, which includes what to eat, when to eat, water therapy, food offering meditation, and conscious eating. The characteristics of a food yogi, the metaphysics of food, sacred foods, the importance of water, the culture of spiritual hospitality – and much more – are explained in detail.

This book is a virtual manifesto of the art and science of food yoga, and is a treasure trove of priceless information about many of the divine aspects of food.

By reading this book you will learn just how important food is to your spiritual journey. You will discover how to genuinely feel compassion and respect for all living beings, and how this universal respect is so fundamental to a food yogi lifestyle.

Foods prepared with loving intention have the ability to unite people in a loving bond. From this excellent book you will learn how to spiritualize your eating, and by doing so, help the world to become a better place.

Kurma Dasa
New Govardhana Farm
Murwillumbah, Australia
14 January 2012
www.kurma.net

INTRODUCTION

Our task must be to free ourselves... widening our circle of compassion to embrace all living creatures and the whole of nature and its beauty. — Albert Einstein.

Just like humans, animals feel pain. Granted, they may not have the intelligence to build a skyscraper, but they do have intelligence, emotions, and are living, breathing, and conscious beings just like we are. Indeed, all things, from insects, to plants, aquatics, and the innumerable single cell organisms that exist everywhere are alive with purpose.

The engine of life is linkage. Everything is linked. Nothing is truly self-sufficient. Just as water and air are inseparable, so too is the interdependence of all living things. We are all united in life for our survival on Earth. Sharing is everything.

This recognition of the oneness of all life is the basis of a truly humane society.

The HOME documentary[2] sums it up this way: "Earth relies on a balance in which every being has a role to play, and exists only through the existence of another being – a subtle, fragile harmony that is easily shattered."

It is the acknowledgement of this interdependence and the need for balance and gratitude that is central to *FOOD YOGA – Nourishing Body, Mind & Soul*.

Our journey begins in the domain of molecular science and quantum physics and establishes the fact that food, like everything in this world, is essentially just another form of energy.

---

[2] *Home* is a 2009 documentary by Yann Arthus-Bertrand. The film is almost entirely composed of aerial shots of various places on Earth. It shows the diversity of life on Earth and how humanity is threatening the ecological balance of the planet.

However this awareness often eludes us humans because we are either too busy consuming food to bother; or we lack the heightened level of sensory perception necessary to notice. This is no more clearly evident than in our embarrassingly poor perception of the electromagnetic spectrum.

Like food, our thoughts are also a form of energy, and therefore they can influence the food we consume, much like conflicting radio waves may scramble a clear signal. When we care more about this powerful influence on our food we will think twice about where we buy our food or where we eat out.

Drawing on numerous mystic traditions, including that of the American Indian, we venture into the esoteric realms of nature spirits and the key role they play in the interplay of energy. This path reveals the sacredness of water and the *pivotal role* it plays in solving the riddle of how to reconnect to our Source.

Although we may not be of this world in spirit, we are certainly bound to it through flesh and the body's concomitant needs. So our journey must, somewhat begrudgingly, take a slight detour to the mundane world of food politics, but makes a strong case for growing our own.

Returning to the central theme of *FOOD YOGA*, we look at the nature of our true self and how we are not only surrounded by energy, but are in essence energetic beings all earnestly seeking the same things: harmony and love.

Having set the framework, we take a deep look at the yoga tradition and how it can help us prosper in body, mind *and* spirit. Yoga is all about connection, but it begins with managing the mind and senses, of which the tongue is the *most* important. How we use our tongues, therefore, is a critical piece of the puzzle.

Since eating is one of the two main functions of the tongue, and so central to our survival, it is logically one of the *most effective* mediums for initiating change in consciousness. Each of us has had the experience of sitting down to a meal cooked with love and felt an immediate transformation of consciousness followed by a feeling of reciprocal love for the person who prepared the meal. The fact is, when food is prepared with loving intention it can communicate in any language. Such food has the ability to break down barriers and turn anger into love, fear into trust, and ignorance into enlightenment. This is no more evident than in the loving exchange between a mother and child.

Unfortunately, although our bodies are hardwired to enjoy eating good food, we often seem bored while eating, distracting ourselves with television, cell phones or the Internet. Even when we are full, we feel unsatisfied and reach for more. American food historian Harvey Levenstein suggests that because of the sheer abundance of food choices in America, there exists a "vague indifference to food, manifested in a tendency to eat and run, rather than to dine and savor."

In FOOD YOGA the case is made that if we make the effort to focus on this very essential part of our lives — eating — incredible and transformative things can happen to us. Biodynamic Guru, Peter Proctor, believes quality food helps people make moral decisions and have moral thoughts — "It's not just stuff to fill your stomach. It actually gives you a real quality of thought and you realize that this is what the world needs."[3]

When you are living consciously, beginning with conscious eating, you will do so in all your thoughts and actions. Your life will be consistent and in harmony with your environment. In other words, you will compliment your environment and not disturb it. Rather than being a "spoke in the wheel" of Nature, you will be a welcome participant in the garden of unlimited possibility.

Food is the most basic necessity of life. Its only purpose is to nourish the body, mind and soul. Food, therefore, should give us life, cleanse our body and uplift our spirit. Eating food

---

[3] Documentary film (2010): *One Man, One Cow, One Planet*

should never be just about fueling the physical body. As Michael Pollan suggests in his book, *In Defense of Food*, "That eating should be foremost about bodily health is a relatively new, and I think, destructive idea - destructive not just of the pleasure of eating, which would be bad enough, but paradoxically of our health as well."

In this context, Pollan specifically refers to the poor health of Americans who are seemingly obsessed with the nutritional content of food at the expense of common sense and happiness. In *FOOD YOGA* we will explore how a more inclusive and respectful attitude toward food and its origins can improve the overall health of your body, mind *and* soul.

According to all yoga traditions, food that is old, decomposed and consisting of dead flesh will pollute the body and consciousness, while food that is fresh, nutritious and free of any suffering will enrich the body, cleanse the mind and satisfy the soul.

The *Bhagavad-gita*[4] states that all foods can be classified according to their inherent quality and the way they affect our body and mind.

> Foods characterized by goodness increase the duration of life, purify one's existence and give strength, health, happiness and satisfaction. Such nourishing foods are sweet, juicy, fattening and palatable.[5]

> Passionate people like foods that are too bitter, too sour, salty, pungent, dry and hot. Such foods cause pain, distress, and disease.[6]

---

[4] *Bhagavad-gita* is a Vedantic scripture comprising the instructions given by Sri Krishna to Arjuna during the Kurukshetra War. It appears as part of the *Mahabharata*.

[5] *Bhagavad-gita As It Is* (17.8) edited for clarity.

[6] *Bhagavad-gita As It Is* (17.9) edited for clarity.

Food cooked more than three hours before being eaten, which is tasteless, stale, putrid, decomposed and unclean, is food liked by unenlightened people.[7]

Foods liked by unenlightened people are essentially those foods that are decomposing and impure. As may be guessed, meat and fish are foods belonging to this lower mode and therefore should be avoided if one truly desires enlightenment and the most sacred connection to the natural world.

Jeremy Rifkin, in his eye-opening chronicling of the meat industry[8] concurs that eating, more than any other single experience, brings us into a full relationship with the natural world.

The act itself calls forth the full embodiment of our senses— taste, smell, touch, hearing, and sight. We know nature largely by the various ways we consume it. Eating establishes the most primordial of all human bonds with the environment, and that is why in most cultures the experience is celebrated as a sacred act and a communion as well as an act of survival and replenishment. Eating, then, is the bridge that connects culture with nature, the social order with the natural order.

Professor Anne Murcott[9] adds, "Food is an especially appropriate 'mediator' because when we eat we establish, in a literal sense, a direct identity between ourselves (culture) and our food (nature)."

In FOOD YOGA we take this concept even further to the point of seeing food as the ultimate peacemaker among all men, animals, and the environment.

---

[7] *Bhagavad-gita As It Is (17.10)* edited for clarity.

[8] *Beyond Beef, the rise and fall of the cattle industry,* Jeremy Rifkin.

[9] *The cultural significance of food and eating.* Proceedings of the Nutrition Society (1982), 41: 203-210 Cambridge University Press.

If we humans honestly recognized the equality of all beings, the collective result would be a desire to share the bounty of the earth and forego all selfish tendencies. The fact that humans do not acknowledge this equality (especially world leaders) is clearly evident in the case of world hunger. *"The problem is not insufficient food production, but inequitable distribution,"* explained UN secretary general, Dr. Kay Killingsworth[10].

Killingsworth made that comment in 1996 and yet here we are in 2012 and world hunger continues to haunt the UN and their Millennium Development Goals (MDG), even though world food production has increased exponentially. How is this possible? I believe the issue is not only inequitable distribution, but also horrendously biased economic policies. For example, can anyone of right mind honestly justify why **35.5% of all grain production in the world is fed to livestock and not humans?**[11] This figure is alarming when we consider that on average, one child dies every five seconds as a result, either directly or indirectly, of hunger – 700 every hour – 16,000 each day - 6 million each year – 60% of all child deaths.[12] In 2012 there should be no hunger whatsoever.

I wonder how many burger-eating Americans and Europeans realize that the majority of this grain is fed to beef cattle grazing on deforested Amazonian lands? According to the FAO[13], the factory farming of animals is *the most* inefficient and environmentally damaging industry in the modern world.

---

[10] United Nations World Food Summit, Rome 1996.

[11] United States Department of Agriculture (USDA) Foreign Agricultural Service (FAS). 2007. Production, Supply & Distribution Online Database. USDA: Washington, D.C. Available online at http://www.fas.usda.gov/psdonline/.

[12] Human Rights Council. *"Resolution 7/14. The right to food"*. United Nations, March 27, 2008, p. 3.

[13] FAO: Food and Agriculture Organization of the United Nations.

Of course, world hunger is a very complex problem, but without doubt, if humans learned to look past racial, religious, ethnic and species differences, there would be no scarcity anywhere in the world. What one entity lacked in its ability to sustain itself, another could contribute through free knowledge, labor exchange, or bartering. It is the symbiotic relationship formed between humans, animals, insects, plants, birds, and fish that have enabled all species to survive throughout the ages.

Unfortunately, the modern capitalist system breeds greed and dishonesty and thus stands in the way of a conscious, sustainable society. Such an ideal society would consist of, what I call *food yogis* or responsible humans that serve, consume, and behave in ways that respect all of creation and help maintain the delicate balance of nature.

Food yogis respect their own body, which they treat as a blessing or a "temple of God." Indeed, they live their entire life in full awareness of their interdependence and interconnectedness to all things. Such a spiritual and all embracing perspective is the foundation of India's *Vedic* culture of hospitality — a culture that is based on the principle of *sama darshana*[14] or spiritual equality.

The *food yogi* fully embraces a socially responsible and environmentally respectful lifestyle. This applies to your choice of food, clothing, cosmetics, cleaning materials and habitat. All should be chosen carefully so that the least amount of harm is inflicted upon your environment and other living things.

This journey in raising consciousness begins with and ends with the tongue. Never underestimate the power of the plate or the power of the spoken word. What you put on your plate is as much a political statement as it is a mirror of who you really are. You can tell much about a person by what comes out of their mouth when they speak and what they consume

---

[14] *Sanskrit: sama:* sameness; *darshinah:* to see.

as food. Food for Life[15] founder Srila Prabhupada[16] often gave the example of a dog on a throne. *"If you throw a shoe, then the dog will leave his throne to chew the shoe,"* he chuckled. Similarly, although an individual may claim to be enlightened or a great moralist, actions speak louder than words, and soon enough those actions will always reveal their true nature.

The Bible says: "The tongue that brings healing is a tree of life, but a deceitful tongue crushes the spirit."[17]

The tongue will always lead the other senses either to purity and thus liberation, or to debauchery and thus perpetual entanglement in sin.

In this spirit, *FOOD YOGA* provides a *Food Offering Meditation* that encapsulates the core lessons learned along the journey, while also respecting the need for the individual to be able to use this meditation within the context of their preferred spiritual tradition. *FOOD YOGA* aims to do this by teaching universally accepted principles of science and spirituality and not dogma.

In *FOOD YOGA*, I also share my personal experiences as a young monk and student of India's Vedic culture of hospitality, while also drawing from numerous scientific and religious sources to provide a believable framework to elevate the act of eating from the shackles of the mundane to the liberating embrace of the transcendental.

---

[15] World's largest plant-based food relief organization. Further reading in Appendix.
[16] A.C. Bhaktivedanta Swami, the founder acharya of ISKCON and scholar who translated and commented on numerous Vedic scriptures.
[17] Proverbs 15:4 NIV.

FOOD YOGA

He who loves with purity considers not the gift of the lover,
but the love of the giver. – *Thomas Kempis*[18]

Rooted in Hindu tradition, the spiritual dimension of food yoga has meaning for people of all faiths. In Hinduism, all food is first offered to God – the very source of that food's creation. Such offerings can be elaborate rituals conducted with great fanfare using expensive paraphernalia and food ingredients, while other offerings may be humble gestures consisting of no more than fresh fruits and water. In all cases, however, it is the intention or the devotion of the aspirant that is foremost. Such offered food is considered pure, karma-free,[19] and spiritually nourishing. Hindus call this food *prasadam,* or the mercy of God.

Hinduism is a complex and varied belief system that accepts many gods and goddesses as emanating from a single source, *Brahman,* which is understood either as an impersonal, formless energy, as in the *Advaita* tradition, or as a dual (male/female) god in the form of *Lakshmi-Vishnu, Radha-Krishna,* or *Shiva-Shakti,* as in *Dvaita* traditions.

To the naturalist, the Goddess is simply "Mother Earth." After all, all food comes from the earth. Some currents of Neopaganism, in particular Wicca, have a concept of a single goddess and a single god who represent a united whole, glorified as the Lord and Lady (*Frey* and *Freya,* literally translated), with the Lord representing abundance and

---

[18] Thomas à Kempis (ca.1380 – 25 July 1471) was a late Medieval Catholic monk and probable author of *The Imitation of Christ,* one of the best-known Christian books on devotion.

[19] Free of any negative reaction resulting from impious behavior.

fertility and the Lady representing peace and love as well as vast powers of magic.

Whatever your belief, the fact that you are reading this book tells me that you may be open to accepting a higher power, and in your own unique way, you honor that higher presence.

My goal here is not to explore the entire subject of foodism, but rather to focus on its more divine aspects, beginning with an acceptance of a benevolent presence in our lives and evolving to appreciating that presence through the offering of pure food, much the same as when you honor a friend in your home. Giving food is the most fundamental act of kindness a human can do, and eating food is one of the few things *all* humans have in common.

Food yoga springs from the belief that the kind of food we eat affects our consciousness and subsequent behaviors. According to the *Bhagavad-gita*, *sattvic*[20] foods can be energetically purified by being offered in devotion, thereby raising one's consciousness. For this reason, food yogis avoid foods saturated with fear and suffering, such as meat, fish, eggs and commercial dairy products,[21] in favor of plant-based meals prepared with loving intention and made with fresh, organic ingredients. Moreover, if people prepare the food you eat with a polluted consciousness (e.g., disgruntled employees working in a dirty restaurant kitchen), you are sure to absorb negative psychic energies.

That food should be prepared and served in its purest possible form is central to the belief and practice of Food for Life Global,[22] a worldwide network of plant-based relief

---

[20] *Sattvic*, Sanskrit word meaning purity. For an object or food to be *sattvic*, it must be physically and energetically pure and lead to clarity and equanimity of mind while also being beneficial to the body.

[21] Unhomogenized and unpasteurized milk that comes from protected cows is considered to be in the mode of goodness.

[22] www.ffl.org

projects. Without adherence to this single principle, Food for Life Global would be no different than any other food relief agency. In fact, the non-profit sees itself more as a social change organization, with pure food as its preferred medium of expression.

At the root of all purity is an adherence to honesty and cleanliness, and both of these attributes can easily be applied to the food industry. The purest food for consumption is food that is energetically pure in *every* phase of its life cycle. When you look beyond the immediate gratification food offers and see food for what it truly is – energy – you tap into one of the greatest wonders of life and open the door to higher awareness.

All the world's great spiritual traditions have elaborate food offering rituals carefully designed to expand consciousness. From the Holy Eucharist to Passover to *Diwali*, Christmas, Thanksgiving, and even the mushroom ceremonies of the Shamanic traditions – all use food as a means to represent or please the Divine and to expand the consciousness of their followers.

Food yoga is, in essence, a discipline that honors all spiritual paths by embracing their core teaching – that food in its most pure form is *divine* and therefore an excellent medium for expressing our unconditional love and purifying our consciousness.

Food yoga is both an art form and a science.

ART: An individual creative expression of love using food as the medium;

SCIENCE: An appreciation for the beauty and interconnectedness of all things, coupled with an unceasing awareness and gratitude for the Energetic Source from which all things emanate.

It's important to create a solid foundation for any belief system, and I propose we break things down to their most elementary level and start by looking at food as nothing more than energy. So let's begin our journey with a little physics.

FOOD AND SCIENCE

What happens to the holes when all the cheese has been eaten?
– Woody Allen.

Food is Energy

The E=MC^2 formula was derived by Albert Einstein in 1905 in one of his *Annus Mirabilis* ("Miraculous Year") papers. One of Einstein's great insights was the realization that matter and energy are really different forms of the same thing. Matter can be turned into energy, and energy into matter.

For example, consider a simple hydrogen atom composed of a single proton.

This subatomic particle has a minute mass of just 0.00000000000000000000000001672 kg.

Taking our example a step further, in one kilogram of pure water there is approximately 111 grams of hydrogen atoms (0.111 kg). Again, a very small number.

However, Einstein's formula reveals the enormous amount of energy this tiny mass of atoms could generate if they were suddenly converted. To calculate the energy (E) of an object, you simply multiply its mass or (M) by the square of the velocity of light^2 or (C). In our example, therefore, the formula would read: 0.111 x 300,000,000 x 300,000,000 = approximately 10,000,000,000,000,000 joules – an incredible amount of energy![23]

A single joule is not a large unit of energy. It is similar to the energy released if you dropped an iPod to the floor. But the amount of potential energy contained in that one

---

[23] The velocity of light is exactly 299,792,458 meters per second; however, it is often approximated as 300,000 kilometers per second or 186,000 miles per second.

kilogram of pure water (10 million, billion joules) is equivalent to 10 million gallons of gasoline!

What Einstein was saying, in effect, was that all matter is really just compressed *energy*, and therefore everything in the universe is ultimately *energy*, including the food we eat. More importantly, from this simple example, you should understand the unlimited energetic potential we all have!

Quantum Physics

Quantum mechanics is a set of scientific principles describing the known behavior of energy and matter that take place at the atomic and subatomic levels.

The "Quantum String Theory" offers that everything in our universe is made up of energies that vibrate at different frequencies.

In *Mysticism and the New Physics*, author Michael Talbot explains that according to modern quantum physics, there is **"no physical world 'out there.'** Consciousness creates all."

"It will be found that both mysticism and the new physics ultimately take the position articulated by Borges in *Other Inquisitions*," writes Talbot. "That is, we have dreamed the world." It is interesting to note that in the description of creation as found in India's *Brahma Samhita*,[24] Lord Maha Vishnu, the source of thousands of avatars and the Creator of countless individual souls, reclines in the waters of the Causal Ocean[25] in a state of divine sleep, called *yoga-nidra* and *dreams* unlimited universes into existence.[26]

---

[24] The *Brahma Samhita* is a Sanskrit *Pancaratra* text, composed of verses of prayer spoken by Brahma glorifying the supreme Lord Krishna or Govinda at the beginning of creation.

[25] The substance from which the material world is created. To initiate the material creation, Maha Vishnu glances at Material Nature, thus agitating her to begin expanding the material elements.

[26] *Brahma Samhita*: Verse 5.47.

English astronomer Sir James Jeans[27] offers the following explanation:

> *Today there is a wide measure of agreement, which on the physical side of science approaches almost to unanimity, that the stream of knowledge is heading towards a non-mechanical reality; the universe begins to look more like a great thought than like a great machine. Mind no longer appears as an accidental intruder into the realm of matter; we are beginning to suspect that we ought rather to hail it as the creator and governor of the realm of matter ...*

Talbot describes this as the "melding of physics and mysticism."

The power of observation

In 1927, German physicist Werner Heisenberg[28] presented his Uncertainty Principle and sparked a debate that to this day has not been resolved. Heisenberg stated that the observer alters the observed by the mere act of the observation.

The problem with observing the minute world of atoms, Heisenberg explained, is that "light profoundly affects them." For example, you take for granted that this page in the book is as you observe it. However, the light reflecting off the page is altering it in a minute way, because in small systems like the interior of an atom, a photon of light actually knocks the particles about. Therefore, we can never pinpoint the exact location of any one particle, since the attempt to do so requires bombarding the particle with photons of light.

What does this mean in a practical sense? Simply that what one perceives, or one's version of reality, *is never* an absolute fact, because matter is constantly reshaping, and, by the mere

---

[27] Sir James Hopwood Jeans OM FRS MA DSc ScD LLD (1877-1946) was an English physicist, astronomer and mathematician.

[28] Werner Heisenberg (1901-1976) was a German theoretical physicist who made foundational contributions to quantum mechanics.

act of observation, things change location. What happens on the subatomic level is far different to what we assume.

Talbot continues, "The discovery that matter is mainly composed of empty space is only the first of many discoveries to destroy the physicists' notions of solid objects on the atomic level." For example it is routinely accepted that 99% of the atom is empty space, or having no measurable matter. That's right, empty! But then how can things feel so solid? Because electrons are negatively charged, when you push your finger against a rock, the electrons in the outer shells of the atoms in your finger will repel the electrons in the outer shells of the atoms in the rock. That's why matter feels so solid – simply because the outer electron shells of atoms repel the outer electron shells of other atoms. *"When you sit on a chair, you are not really touching it."* [29]

New Zealand physicist Ernest Rutherford's[30] experiments confirmed that matter consists mainly of vast empty regions of space filled with energy in the form of particles or waves. "Depending on how we look at it, a subatomic entity displays the properties of both a particle and a wave," explains Talbot.

Talbot then offers that with Heisenberg's proposal that physicists should simply accept the paradoxical aspect of subatomic entities and view them as waves/particles, Heisenberg was in essence **"making a statement that belonged as much to mysticism as it did to the new physics,"** or that the nature of reality was *"beyond verbal description."*

While there is much we still don't understand about the universe, the most important concept to grasp is that everything is interconnected. For example, if we could freeze time just before the so-called "Big Bang," we would see that for a brief instant only one common energy existed.

---

[29] http://education.jlab.org/qa/atomicstructure_10.html
[30] Ernest Rutherford, First Baron Rutherford of Nelson, OM, FRS (1871-1937) was a New Zealand chemist and physicist who became known as the father of nuclear physics.

Everything in the universe emanated from that singular energetic event. Whether we accept that in the beginning, the universe was created by a great cataclysm, or by the seed of a pure sound, as in the name of God, it makes no difference because ultimately in both scenarios, energy is the clear impetus. Every tangible thing we experience in this universe, whether it be mountains, trees, insects, fish, animals, humans, planets, or galaxies, etc., are in essence different forms of the same stuff which stars are made of.

Interconnectedness

This became clearly apparent in 1967, when Pulsars were discovered. Pulsars are neutron stars that emit regular *pulses* of electromagnetic waves. They are formed from the explosion of supernovas[31], from which all elements of matter are derived. Inevitably, some of the matter from these supernova explosions are pulled into the earths gravitational field. It's estimated that hundreds of millions of tons of such mineral-rich "stardust" falls onto the earth every year, and in one way or another, becomes the fruits, vegetables, nuts, seeds and grains we eat.

Everything in the universe shares an energetic familiarity. Therefore, like a domino effect, any change in this universal web of interconnectedness affects everything else. This interconnectedness explains our ability to influence the lives of others, and how thoughts affect food.

Thoughts and Emotions are Energy

People are starting to realize that thoughts are energy, too, and over the last two decades, we've seen an explosion of self-help books like *The Secret* by Robyn Byrne, all essentially stating one simple message: positive thinking leads to a more fulfilling life. "The first step to using the *Law of Attraction*,"

---

[31] A supernova is a stellar explosion that is so luminous that the burst of radiation often briefly outshines an entire galaxy!

says Byrne, is "to clarify exactly what you want," because "thoughts are things." The vibration you radiate to the universe is comprised of your thoughts, emotions, and actions.

What you think about and the strength of the emotions you attach to that thing will either attract what *you want* or attract what you *don't want*. If you are constantly meditating on your past failures and poor health, you can expect more of the same. Conversely, if you focus your attention on health and prosperity, you can expect as such. In other words, your thoughts are literally writing the "screenplay" of your life.

Shakti Gawain, a pioneer in the field of personal development and the best-selling author of numerous books, including *Creative Visualization*, explains how to use mental imagery and affirmations to produce positive changes in one's life. Her book contains meditations and exercises to help practitioners channel their energies in positive directions. For example, she recommends having a regular creative visualization meditation period for fifteen minutes each morning upon arising, and each evening just before sleep, as these are the times when it is most effective. She suggests, "always starting your meditation periods with deep relaxation, then following with any visualizations or affirmations you wish."

Not surprisingly, some of the world's leading scientists in physics, biology, psychology and many other fields are starting to recognize the importance of thought energy. In fact, positive thought energy in the form of collective meditation has already been scientifically proven to reduce violent crime!

Intention experiment

In 1993, one of the world's leading physicists proposed a study to determine if the focused meditation of a large group of participants in Transcendental Meditation® and TM-Sidhi could have an effect on Washington DC's crime rate. The results were astonishing.

The official report from the Institute of Science

Technology and Public Policy states:

> Based on the results of the study, the steady state gain (long-term effect) associated with a permanent group of 4,000 participants in the Transcendental Meditation and TM-Sidhi programs was calculated as a 48% reduction in HRA crimes in the District of Columbia.
>
> Given the strength of these results, their consistency with the positive results of previous research, the grave human and financial costs of violent crime, and the lack of other effective and scientific methods to reduce crime, policy makers are urged to apply this approach on a large scale for the benefit of society.[32]

This scientifically validated method of countering the criminal inclinations of a very large city proves beyond a doubt that thought, and specifically focused intention, is a form of energy that can affect the world around us.

Lynn McTaggart, author of *The Intention Experiment* documents hundreds of examples of the effects of group focused intention in scientifically controlled experiments.

Leaf glow

On March 11, 2007, Lynn McTaggert and her team carried out a test using the attendees of an Intention Experiment conference held by her publishing company in London. Her assistant Mark Boccuzzi, operating remotely, set up a webcam and live images of two geranium leaves to broadcast on their website, visible only to Lynne and her London audience. In order to achieve statistical significance, Lynn felt she needed more than thirty data points with which

[32] Reference: Hagelin, J.S., Rainforth, M.V., Orme-Johnson, D.W., Cavanaugh, K. L., Alexander, C.N., Shatkin, S.F., Davies, J.L, Hughes, A.O, and Ross, E. 1999. Effects of group practice of the Transcendental Meditation program on preventing violent crime in Washington D.C.: Results of the National Demonstration Project, June-July, 1993. Social Indicators Research, 47(2): 153-201.

to compare the two leaves. Psychologist Dr. Gary Schwartz, director of the Center for Advances in Consciousness and Health, was asked to puncture each leaf sixteen times.

Although the participants would know the target leaf, the scientists would not be told until they'd calculated the results.

A member of the audience was then asked to choose the target leaf by flipping a coin, at which time the chosen leaf was displayed on a projector. After engaging the audience in a simple "Powering Up" exercise, the group held a focused intention to make the leaf glow for 10 minutes.

The remote scientists were only told which leaf had been chosen after they'd finished their calculations. A week later, Dr. Schwartz revealed that the changes in the light emissions of the leaf given the glowing intention had been so strong that they could readily be seen in the digital images created by the CCD cameras.

Apparently, the increased biophoton effect was highly statistically significant and that, "all the punctured holes in the chosen leaf were filled with light." All the holes in the control leaf, on the other hand, remained black.

Other Worlds

All the world's spiritual traditions tell us that there are multiple dimensions existing right now in the world in which we live. Due to the limitation of our human senses, we are not able to perceive these other worlds, but it wasn't always that way.

Many of us can attest that when we were children, we were able to perceive these other worlds. Whether this was the result of gullible innocence, purity, openness, or our senses being less frazzled by the modern lifestyle, it is hard to know for sure. But I can still remember the morning when I first saw otherworldly beings standing in my room.

I was about 6 years old when I suddenly awoke around 5AM to find a man and a woman standing near the door looking at me. They were wearing white robes and seemed harmless in nature, but I wondered why they were there. In a state of confusion, I covered my face with the blankets and prayed. I have no recollection of what happened after that. Later that morning I told my mother about my "visitors." Probably because she didn't want to alarm me, she responded, "Oh, don't worry, son, it is only your imagination." My little brain tried hard to comprehend this new big word, "imagination," but I really couldn't understand. Rather than challenge my mother, however, I accepted her explanation and went about playing again. Now, some 40 years later, as I vividly recall those two people standing in my room, I can't discount that experience as a mere figment of my imagination. There *were* people in my room that morning, although I have no idea who they were or why they were there in the first place.

Suffice to say that I am convinced, as you most probably are, that what we see with these physical eyes during our normal daily activities is by no means a complete picture of the world we live in. In fact, science fully verifies this.

Electromagnetic Spectrum

The electromagnetic spectrum is the range of all possible frequencies of electromagnetic radiation. An object's electromagnetic spectrum is the characteristic distribution of electromagnetic radiation emitted or absorbed by that particular object.

The electromagnetic spectrum (EM) extends from below frequencies used for modern radio to gamma radiation at the short wavelength end, covering wavelengths from thousands of kilometers down to a fraction of the size of an atom.

Electromagnetic radiation that can be detected by the human eye is called *visible light*. Within the electromagnetic spectrum, a typical human eye will respond to wavelengths from about 380 to 750 nm[33]. The entire electromagnetic spectrum ranges from 10 megameters to a very minute 1 picometer. In layman's terms, this means that more than 99% of the total electromagnetic spectrum is completely beyond our ability to perceive it! Think about that for a second. *Human eyes can only perceive about 1% of the entire electromagnetic spectrum* yet, somewhat audaciously, we hold onto the notion that "seeing is believing."

We often see this in modern science, where theories on creation and the nature of the universe are posited, only to be retracted or adjusted according to newer discoveries or academic bullying. Textbooks are constantly being rewritten. One of the great dilemmas for modern physicists in piecing together the puzzle of creation is rationalizing what they propose to be an accurate picture, with the fact that so many pieces of the puzzle cannot be found.

Dark Energy

However, there are no shortages of theories among physicists to explain the universe and its contents. One such theory to explain the so-called "missing mass" in the universe is the "dark energy" and "dark matter" theories.

The quest to solve the puzzle of whether "dark matter" or "dark energy" exists and, if so, what it consists of is extremely important to the scientific world, and for good reason. Because without this confirmation, all their other theories are useless.

According to the theory, although this dark matter is invisible and emits no electromagnetic radiation, it *must* have a large cumulative mass since its presence is measurable through its gravitational effects on visible matter. "Dark energy" is simply the remaining unknown. The standard

---

[33] (nm) Nanometer is a unit of spatial measurement equating to one billionth of a meter. It is commonly used in nanotechnology, the building of extremely small machines.

model of cosmology theorizes that dark matter and dark energy accounts for around 95%[34] of all existence in the Universe.

So let's make this simple: this means that about 95% of the universe is unknown! That's right, the greatest minds on our planet with access to the most advanced technology, cannot say, with absolute certainty, what 95% of the puzzle of life is. Therefore, creating any kind of theory under these circumstances is sort of like attempting to create an encyclopedia on a scrabble board without knowing what letters even exist in the box!

Oddly enough, there is a striking correlation between the dark matter, dark energy theories being proposed today and the teachings of Eastern mystics, who suggest that there exists an energetic 'field' that connects all things in this universe and that this energy, known as the *Brahman-jyotir* emanates from Visnu. The word *Brahman* literally means "spiritual," and *jyotir* means "light." According to the *Bhagavad-gita*[35], everything that exists is situated within the all-pervasive light energy (*brahma-jyotir*) of Visnu. However, when this *brahma-jyotir* is covered by illusion, it is called "material energy", in the same way that a shadow is created when we turn our back to a light source.

The Superior Senses of Animals

Many animals have far superior senses, and some species can see wavelengths that fall outside humans' visible spectrum. Bees and other insects, for example, can see light into the ultraviolet range, which helps them find nectar in flowers.

---

[34] The WMAP (Wilkinson Microwave Anisotropy Probe) seven-year analysis gave an estimate of 72.8% dark energy, 22.7% dark matter and 4.6% ordinary matter.

[35] *Bhagavad-gita As it is*, Verse: 4.24

Plant species that depend on insect pollination may owe reproductive success to their appearance in ultraviolet light, rather than how colorful they appear to us.

For example, the rising sun's light filtered by the atmosphere appears to us as red, however, insects like bees are blind to this color. Whereas, our color vision is sensitive to green, blue and red, the bees are sensitive to green, blue and ultraviolet. With only three basic colors, we both create a full color picture, however, the bees worldview is a lot more courser. Seen through a bee's eye, flowers become strangely unfamiliar. For example, the pretty yellow buttercup flower looks more pink. But maybe this is the true color, because the colors we see have no real relevance to the flower's evolution. For the flower, these hidden hues have evolved to attract insects.

Birds have the most complex color vision of any animal. They can see well into the ultraviolet range (300-400 nm), and some have sex-dependent markings on their plumage that are only visible in the ultraviolet range. The light sensitive cells of the bird's eye contain up to five different color pigments. These pigments detect many more color hues than we can see. While the cells of the eye also contain colored oil droplets that act like miniature filters and reveal even more colors! The eyesight of birds such as eagles, hawks and buzzards is 3-4 times sharper than ours. Eagles can spot rabbits from several miles away while hawks and buzzards often scan the earth from a height of 10-15,000 feet looking for tasty rodents! And when they spot one, these birds can dive at over 100 mph and still keep their target in complete focus.

Other examples of the superior senses of animals are a dog's ability to hear sounds over a wider range of frequencies and a greater distance than we can. Experiments have shown that an average dog can locate the source of a sound in about six-hundredths of a second. Similarly, a wolf has a sense of smell, 100 times sharper than that of human beings, and possess a staggering 200 million olfactory cells in their nose.

Most impressively, a spider can weave a web that has greater tensile strength than steel; an ant can lift up to 50 times its body weight, and the Monarch butterfly's annual migration has been described as the most astonishing example of endurance in the natural world. Monarchs use a combination of air currents and thermals to travel as far as 3,000 miles to reach their winter home.

The list of amazing feats within the non-human world goes on and on. The fact is, when it comes to vision, endurance, strength, hearing, smelling or dexterity, we human-animals can't compete. We simply do not have the physical capacity to fully fathom the depths of the known world.

But then how is it, that some humans can have moments of higher perception? Mystic traditions are laden with stories of humans possessing supernatural sensual abilities, and there are also many documented cases in recent history of humans being able to literally see and record events taking place in distant places using a technique called "remote viewing.[36]"

It appears that with practice, humans can develop higher sense perception. However, it could also be argued that if society at large curtailed its addiction to intoxication in all its forms, along with the mind numbing effects of television, radio, newspapers and live sport, we may naturally expand our awareness as a result of life experiences. Sadly, though, whereas age is meant to be synonymous with wisdom, in most cases, it becomes an embarrassingly harsh footnote to a wasted human life.

---

[36] Remote viewing is the ability to gather information about a distant or unseen target using paranormal means, in particular, extra-sensory perception (ESP) or sensing with the mind alone. From World War II until the 1970s the US government funded ESP research, and many believe that psychic enhancement programs continue to be a formidable part of modern US military strategy.

There is much to learn in this respect from the indigenous traditions of the world.

METAPHYSICS

The worst sin towards our fellow creatures is not to hate them, but to be indifferent to them, that's the essence of inhumanity. – Isaac Bashevis Singer

American Indians

The American Indians, also known as the "People of the Land," have traditionally and historically held "a special knowledge of the land and its inhabitants," explains, Takatoka, of the Manataka American Indian Council. Such intimate knowledge and thus a higher sensitivity to the world around them was possible, he suggests, "because of a belief system that considered all things of creation equal, essential, and worthy of respect."

This belief system has been enormously beneficial to the world, he claims, because "most of the world's pharmacopoeia (healing medicines) can be traced back to Native Americans' tremendous knowledge of the plant kingdom." American Indians' knowledge of herbal medicine, healing stones, healing clay, and animal wisdom is on par with, if not superior to, many of the world's greatest civilizations.

Although there are over five hundred American Indian tribes, the universal beliefs they share transcend ethnic, cultural and geographic boundaries.

Takatoka explains that common among those traditional teachings are the following basic beliefs:

- Never take more than we need.
- Thank the Creator for what we have or what we will receive.
- Use all of what we have.
- Give away what we do not need.

Because American Indians respect Nature, they kill only what they need to survive. They do not waste life, but use every part of the sacrificed animal. After the kill, they pray to their spirit guides to lead them to the slain animal's spirit so

43

they may personally thank the spirit; they then honor the soul by leaving a gift where the animal fell.

American Indians traditionally give special recognition to the power of the animal spirits by wearing the animal skin and feathers in ceremonial dance. They often paint pictures of the animals on their bodies and carry parts of the animals in their medicine bags. Such practices allow American Indians to remain connected to the animal guides so the animals may teach them their powers and impart spiritual wisdom. All these conscientious acts help remind the American Indians that all things in creation are their brothers, sisters, cousins, and more importantly teachers and friends. They believe that humans are also animal spirits.

"American Indians view all things in creation as having spiritual energy," says Takatoka. We see "all things as connected," and therefore "worthy of our respect and reverence." Their path is to continually seek balance and harmony within the complex tapestry called the "Great Circle of Life."

John Robbins wrote about the connectedness of the American Indians in his book, *Diet for a New America* (1987):

> *The Indians who dwelt for countless centuries in what we now call the United States lived in harmony with the land and with nature. Their societies were each unique, yet all were founded on a reverence for life that conserved nature rather than destroying it, and which lived in balance with what we today call the ecosystem. To them, it was all the work of God. Every shining pine needle, every sandy shore, every mist in the dark woods, every humming insect was holy.*

When the crusading white men forced them to sell their land, their leader, Chief Seattle, did not ask for any personal benedictions for himself or his people, but instead asked only one thing in return. His humble and selfless request was prophetic as it was plain:

I will make one condition. The white man must treat the beasts of this land as his brothers. For whatever happens to the beasts soon happens to man. All things are connected.

Sadly, the white leaders of the time considered the Chief and his people as ignorant savages and yet his wise words are strikingly similar to the Holy Bible that the white men hailed as the word of God.

For that which befalleth the sons of men befalleth the beasts. Even one thing befalleth them: as the one dieth, so dieth the other; yea they have all one breath, so that a man hath no pre-eminence above a beast.[37]

Although the Chief had no knowledge of the Bible, his words of advice to the white men were almost identical:

One thing we know; our God is the same, this earth is precious to Him ...

This we know: The earth does not belong to man: Man belongs to the earth.

This we know: All things are connected, like the blood, which unites one family.

All things are connected. Whatever befalls the earth befalls the sons of the earth. Man did not weave the web of life. He is merely a strand in it. Whatever he does to the web, he does to himself.

American Indians essentially emphasize the following truths:
- Everything on earth is alive.
- Everything on earth has purpose.
- Everything on earth is connected.
- Everything on earth is to be embraced.

---

[37] *Ecclesiastes* 3:19.

Native Americans believe that all things on Earth and all things in the universe are capable of being spirit guides. Why? "Because the spirit of the Creator is in all things," they say.

The Personification of Nature

We should not be surprised by references to spirit guides within nature. From time immemorial, humans have personified their awe and reverence for the wonders of the Universe. To many, these references are simply symbolic or metaphor; however, a closer look at the great spiritual traditions of the world reveal a logical and common sense portrayal of these wonders.

All around us we see amazing displays of ingenuity, creativity, and adaptation. Such traits are necessary if one wishes to endure and succeed in any endeavor. These qualities are essentially personal. We never see such diverse and innovative brilliance displayed by inanimate things. Only animate beings possessing personal traits have such capacity.

Take a watch for example: It comprises hundreds of tiny pieces all expertly arranged to create, not only a timepiece, but also a work of art. Now, if we were to take these individual pieces and place them in a box, shake the box and then throw the pieces onto a table, is it even remotely possible that these watch parts will assemble themselves into that same work of art? Of course not. But essentially, this is the same illogical reasoning being used to support the impersonal mechanistic view of the Universe. A belief system that proposes that by chance alone all the ingredients of nature came together to magically form complex life forms!

Intelligent Design

In a brazen effort to explain Darwin's evolutionary theory, biochemist Dean Kenyan released a book called *Biochemical Predestination* in 1969, proposing that proteins could assemble themselves into ordered life forms.

However, five years after its publication, Kenyan began doubting his theory. Upon further review into the nature of proteins, he and the scientific community became aware that without the *instructional code* of DNA it was impossible for proteins to self-assemble.

"The more I conducted my own studies ... the more it became apparent that there were multiple difficulties with the chemical evolution account, and further experiments showed that amino acids do not have the ability to order themselves into any meaningful biological sequences."

The more Kenyan pondered the key role of DNA, the new question became, "Where do these genetic assembly instructions of DNA come from?

"If one could find the origin of the encoded messages within the living machinery, then you'd really be onto something far more intellectually satisfying than this chemical evolution theory," he suggests.

Indeed, the expanding body of knowledge about DNA is a goldmine for proponents of Intelligent Design. By the late 1970s, most researchers had rejected the idea that the information needed to build the first cell originated by chance alone. To better understand why, consider the foolishness of trying to create even a simple five-letter word in a game of Scrabble by dropping the letters onto the board. Then consider that the specific **genetic instructions required to build a simple one cell organism would fill hundreds of pages of printed text!**

In other words, just like the content of a book cannot be explained by the paper and ink that it is made of, so too the content of the genetic code cannot be explained by any set of natural forces. The critical role of DNA instructional codes requires biologists to make a determination about origins.

The creationist view of the universe, however, accepts a divine intelligence or Supreme Creator as the most logical explanation for the source of DNA instructional codes and other wonders of the universe. Contrary to atheistic claims, this view is not based exclusively on faith, for one can just as easily arrive at this same conclusion using logic.

Everything in our world, whether it is the book you hold now; the iPad you use; the house you reside in; or the car you drive - every single one of them became a reality because of some person or persons designing and creating it. There are absolutely no exceptions to this rule. Then why is it so difficult to accept that the universe and all its astonishing diversity and complexity came to be because of an even far greater personified Designer and Creator?

We see, feel, hear, touch and smell personality everywhere; it is logical to conclude, therefore, that the same personal characteristic exists throughout the universe and that personality is the basis of all creation.

This begs the question: Who created the original personality? A similar question was raised by the crew in the movie *Promethius*[38] when they contemplated the possibility that humans were seeded by an alien life form. "Who created them?" one of the crew asked. Of course, these "chicken or the egg" debates on who or what started this whole cosmic creation are bound by the limitations of time. Time is the great equalizer; the great controller of this world. No one escapes the influence of time. Where there is the influence of time, there must be a beginning and an end. By definition, the event becomes measurable in time units and therefore we think in linear terms. But what if time was cyclical? What if the energy of this world always existed, but only changed shape over time? What if time was an illusion? Time is certainly relative. What we experience to be a significant length of time is insignificant to the life of a planet. Similarly, the entire life of a moth is only about 24 hours of human time. What if time was only influential on the more denser

---

[38] *Prometheus* is a 2012 American science fiction film directed by Ridley Scott, and is a prequel to the 1979 film *Alien*.

levels of creation, and that in the higher realms it ceased to exist, or was conspicuous by its absence, as the Vedas suggest?

The concept of a personal God is prevalent throughout all spiritual traditions and this same God-like force is portrayed as unlimited, omniscient, and beyond the control of time, or eternal. Once we factor in the possibility that the ultimate creative force is not bound by time, the dilemma of who or what was the original seed of existence becomes a moot point.

Animism

An example of the personification of the universe can be found in the Animism traditions of the world that hold that all non-human entities are spiritual beings, and that inanimate objects like mountains and rivers embody some kind of personified life-principle.

This idea is certainly not exclusive to Native American tradition, but can also be seen in African traditional religions, the Shinto traditions of Japan, some forms of Hinduism, Sikhism, Buddhism, Pantheism, Islam, Modern Neopaganism, and Wicca. Furthermore, throughout European history, philosophers such as Aristotle and Thomas Aquinas,[39] the model of Catholic priesthood, contemplated the possibility that souls exist in animals, plants, and people. Moreover, the American holiday of Thanksgiving has an address by the Iroquois tribe which is filled with praises for every being, beginning with the Mother Earth, the waters, fish, plants, herbs, animals, trees, birds, winds, thunders, Brother sun, Grandmother Moon, stars, enlightened teachers and finally God.[40]

---

[39] Thomas Aquinas, (1225-1274) was an Italian Dominican priest of the Catholic Church, and an immensely influential philosopher and theologian.

[40] *The Iroquois Thanksgiving Address*: The Iroquois, also known as the *Haudenosaunee* or the "People of the Longhouse", are an association of several tribes of indigenous people of North America.

Animism is based on the belief that personal life force abounds everywhere; that the spiritual and physical worlds overlap, and that souls or spirits exist in all animals, plants, rocks, and even natural phenomena such as lightning, mountains and rivers.

In the Vedic traditions of India, personified Nature Devas are believed to be responsible for managing the elements of nature, namely, fire (lightning), air (wind), water (rain) and earth (trees). Whereas the more powerful Devas (Mahadevas) like Agni, Vayu, and Indra control the provision of those elements and the intricate tasks governing the functioning of the cosmos.

Nature Devas and Mahadevas, however, are not to be confused with the Supreme Personality of Godhead. The *Bhagavat Purana* explains:

> *Out of fear of the Supreme Personality of Godhead the wind blows, the sun shines, the rain pours forth showers, and the host of heavenly bodies shed their luster.* [41]

Since earth, water, fire, and air are all essential elements in the growing of food, it is important to be appreciative of these "caretakers of nature". We do this by respecting our environment and doing whatever is necessary to conserve nature.

However, in a world that is so dominated by the male energy of fire, as evidenced in the proliferation of industry, cities and wars, etc., the nurturing, healing, and feminine qualities of water are more critical than ever to the survival of our species. Ironically, and sadly, many pundits believe future wars will be fought over water.

Our research into the divinity of food, therefore, continues with a thought-provoking analysis of this most important element.

---

[41] *Bhagavat Purana* Verse 3.29.40

WATER

Water is life's mater and matrix, mother and medium.
There is no life without water. – Albert Szent-Gyorgyi [42]

Human bodies are composed of approximately 90% water at birth and about 60% water as adults. Throughout our lives, we rely on water to hydrate and purify our bodies and to aid in digestion and other bodily functions that keep us alive. In ritual, water is used to baptize and to rebirth a person; in the form of steam, it draws toxins from the body, and as ice it cools and preserves. In a world that is becoming physically drier and increasingly characterized by human insensitivity, greed and stubbornness, water's flexibility, tenderness and ability to sustain life symbolize the cure for all.

Water is the primary energizer of every function of the body. Where there are empty spaces in the body there is primarily water. It is the transportation vehicle for blood circulation and the adhesive that binds the solid parts of a cell together. Similar to ice in its tackiness, water seems to become sticky at the cell membrane and thus it helps in holding things together and forming a protective barrier around the cell.

The neurotransmission systems of the brain and nerves depend on the rapid movement of sodium and potassium in and out of the cell membrane along the full length of the nervous system and water plays a critical role. Water that is unengaged in the nerve tissues, or in other words, not bonded with something else, is able to freely move across the cell membrane and turn the "voltage-generating pumps" of the cell, thus generating energy and forcing potassium into the

---

[42] Albert Szent-Gyorgyi (Hungarian Biochemist, 1937 Nobel Prize for Medicine, 1893-1986).

cell while pushing sodium outside the cell. It is this surge of *excess* water that creates hydroelectric energy in the body.

This molecular process in the micro universe is similar to how the force of water turns the turbines at a hydroelectric dam to generate electricity in the macro universe. Most people assume that the intake of food alone is the sole reason why there is "heat" in the stomach to "cook" or digest food, and the fuel needed for the numerous other chemical reactions required for the cells to function. Modern biological research, however, now confirms that in fact *water* is the central regulator of energy and osmotic[43] balance in the body. Moreover, there is significant evidence, particularly in the research of Fereydoon Batmanghelidj[44], suggesting that the primary cause of osteoporosis and a host of other modern ailments is not calcium deficiency but rather chronic dehydration.

All the food we eat is a product of energy conversion from the initial electrical-energy-generating property of water. *All living and growing species survive as a result of the energy generated by water.*

A lack of understanding for the magnitude of our body's dependence on energy generated from cellular hydroelectricity is a major problem in allopathic evaluations of the body.

For example, when the body is fully hydrated, blood is normally about 94% water. In this state, the red blood cells become like "water bags" containing the red-colored

---

[43] *Osmosis:* Diffusion of fluid through a semipermeable membrane from a solution with a low solute concentration to a solution with a higher solute concentration until there is an equal concentration of fluid on both sides of the membrane.

[44] Fereydoon Batmanghelidj (1931 – November 15, 2004) was born in Tehran, Iran. He was best known for his book, *Your Body's Many Cries for Water*, and his writings related to health and wellness.

hemoglobin. For optimum health, the cells of our body should ideally contain on average about 75% water.

Only *excess* or unengaged water can move about and thus generate hydroelectric energy at the cell membrane. The already existing water inside the body will be engaged with all other functions for life support. It follows then that fresh, clean water should be consumed at regular intervals throughout the day and therefore must be considered the ultimate restorative beverage.

How Much Water Should I Drink?

The Mayo Clinic[45] advises that men should consume roughly 3 liters (about 13 cups) of non-diuretic drinks a day and women around 2.2 liters (about 9 cups) of total per day.

Another rule of thumb is to consume about 1 liter of clean water per 30kgs of body weight. Essentially you should drink enough water so that you never feel thirsty, your mouth never becomes dry, and you can produce about 1.5 liters (6.3 cups) or more of colorless urine throughout the day.

You might think it's impractical to consume so much water; however, a good way to get your daily water requirement is to adopt the food yogi morning rehydration ritual. The body is naturally acidic and dehydrated in the morning, having fasted from water and food for 6–8 hours. The best way to break our night fast, therefore, is not with acidifying toast and coffee, but with highly alkaline spring water. Bread is acidic and drying and so it will make our body even more dehydrated, and since coffee is an acidic beverage it too will increase the body's acidity and facilitate disease. It is best to keep the body slightly alkaline pH[46] in order to

---

[45] A not-for-profit medical practice and medical research in the United States.

[46] pH is a scale that measures how acidic or alkaline a substance is. The scale ranges from 1 to 14 with 1 being very acid, 7 neutral and 14 very alkaline.

maintain optimum health. Why is this important? There are two factors always present with cancer and all other diseases: acidic pH levels in the body and a lack of oxygen.

An acidic pH level can result from an acid-forming diet, stress, toxic overload, lack of nutrients, or any situation that deprives your cells of fresh oxygen. The ideal pH level for your blood is around 7.35. The body will always try to compensate for acidic pH by using alkaline minerals stored in your body, because if your blood pH were to vary 1 or 2 points in either direction, the electrical chemistry within your body would shut down, leading to death. If your diet does not contain enough minerals, a build up of acids in the cells will occur.

The best way to avoid upsetting this delicate bio chemical balance is to consume an alkaline diet and to drink alkaline water, thus ensuring your red blood cells can deliver oxygen and nutrients throughout your body as efficiently as possible. It is important to understand that it isn't how "acid" something tastes when you eat or drink it, but rather; what the pH reaction is within the body when you digest it. For example, citrus fruits like lemons create an alkaline reaction in the body. Most of the things people consume these days creates an acidic reaction. These include alcohol, coffee, tea, processed foods, and animal proteins.

All green vegetables have an alkaline reaction on the body, and therefore a convenient way to begin changing your pH from acidic to slightly alkaline is to drink "green drinks" by adding green powders like barley grass to your fresh juices. Live bodies need live, wholesome, alkaline green foods for optimum health. However, alkaline waters are *the most* effective in addressing acidosis (increased acidity in the blood) because with water there is no added waste product. Alkaline water with any diet will do wonders.

Research has proven that diseases cannot survive in an alkaline state and yet they thrive in an acidic environment. Dr. George W. Crile, past head of the Crile Clinic in

Cleveland, US and a recognized surgeon believes acidosis precedes and provokes disease: "There is no natural death. All deaths from so-called natural causes are merely the end-point of a progressive acid saturation."

Although we may have different nutritional needs, there is one thing we all have in common — we need to have alkaline blood to stay healthy.

Food Yogi Rehydration Method

The following routine will get you well on the way to creating a healthy, vibrant, alkaline body. As soon as you wake up and have passed urine, open the window and take three deep breaths and expend all the stale air out of your lungs by filling them with fresh morning air.

Next, cleanse your tongue with a spoon to remove the mucus that has accumulated overnight (do not brush your teeth yet) and then drink 1 to 1.5 liters of pure spring water with a pH level of at least 7.4. For extra value, add the freshly squeezed juice of one lemon to increase the electrolyte content and cleansing power of the water. It should take you about 20 - 30 minutes to drink this amount. After completing the water, brush your teeth but do not eat anything for at least 60 minutes, or until you have passed the majority of this water out of your system. By the time you pass urine for the 2nd and 3rd time your urine should be very clear and odorless. After breakfast, lunch and dinner do not drink anything for at least one hour. Between meals continue to sip small amounts at a time to keep your mouth moist. If you like to drink some fluid during a meal, make sure it is hot or warm and very little - just enough to aid digestion. You don't want to "flood" the stomach and thus destroy the digestive process.

By consuming a large amount of water first thing in the morning our body remains in a hydrated state throughout the day, and will only require small top-ups to supply the body with enough "unengaged" water to keep the system working optimally.

The morning hydration routine has been known to help with a number of ailments, including high blood pressure, diabetes, constipation, migraine, arthritis and many stomach problems.

The treatment has no side effects, but during the initial stages of the treatment you might find yourself urinating more than you're used to.

If you're concerned about your fluid intake, check with your doctor or a registered dietitian. They can help you determine the amount of water that's best for you.

Most people will say they never feel thirsty enough to drink so much water, but Dr. Batmandhelidj believes that through years of chronic dehydration a person loses their sense of thirst. In other words, they begin to interpret the body's cry for water as a signal of hunger and thus they mistakenly snack instead of drinking water.

The superiority of water, as opposed to other beverages, as a source of energy, is the fact that any excess water is always passed out of the body. Using this excess water, the body manufactures the necessary energy to stock up the reserves in the cells and then easily expels it, sending with it all the toxic waste of the cells.

In cases where a person is not drinking sufficient water throughout the day, the cells become depleted of their available energy, resulting in a dependence on energy generated from food. The body is then forced into storing fat and using its protein and starch reserves, because they are easier to break down than stored fat. Besides an unhealthy diet and inactivity, this is a critical reason why over 25%[47] of

---

[47] Source: The Centers for Disease Control and Prevention (CDC) reports that 42 states in the US had a prevalence equal to or greater than 25%. www.cdc.gov

people in America are obese[48]. Their bodies are in a constant crisis of dehydration management.

The process of hydrolysis denotes that water is involved in the metabolism of other materials. The breaking down of protein into the different amino acids and the breakdown of large fatty particles into smaller fatty acid units require hydrolysis. Without water, hydrolysis cannot take place. We can conclude, therefore, that the hydrolytic[49] function of water must also constitute the metabolism of water itself. Translation: water also needs to be broken down or hydrolyzed before the body can use the various components in food and hence; the critical need to supply the body with ample clean water well before we eat solid foods.

Sacred Waters

In places like India, water is regarded as a sentient being, revered and personified as an aspect of divinity. The Ganges River is worshiped by hundreds of millions of Indians daily. Indeed, water is prayed to and worshiped in many traditions, and yet the modern industrial machine chooses to ignore this fact and wreaks havoc on the world's water systems.

We can only imagine how beautiful and pure the Earth's eco-systems were when ancient civilizations held reverence for water as a sacred, integral element of their lives and there were no pharmaceutical plants and slaughterhouses upstream, spewing out disgusting waste.

Water plays an essential role in the story of creation. The *Koran* states, "From water we have made all things." According to Greek mythology, *hydros* (or Hydrus) was the protogenos of the primordial waters. In the *Orphic Theogonies*,

---

[48] Obesity is defined as a body mass index (BMI) of 30 or greater.

[49] Hydrolytic: Decomposition of a chemical compound by reaction with water, such as the dissociation of a dissolved salt or the catalytic conversion of starch to glucose.

Water was the first being to emerge at creation alongside Creation (*Thesis*) and Mud. The primordial mud solidified into *Gaia* (Earth) and with *Hydros*, produced *Khronos* (Time) and *Ananke* (Compulsion). These two in turn caught the early cosmos in the coils, and split it apart to form the God Phanes (creator of life), as well as the four ordered elements of Heaven (Fire), Earth, Air and Sea (Water)[50].

Internationally renowned voice coach, Stewart Pearce[51] points out that the word "human" is "drawn from the ancient words connected with the spirit of God....The sound *hu* in the word "human" means "the breath of spirit" (*Sanskrit*), while *mah* means "water" (*Arabic*). The Bible says: "*Except a man be born of water and spirit, he cannot enter into the Kingdom of heaven.*"

The *Bhagavata Purana*[52] contains an elaborate description of creation, including the unfolding of the five principle elements, earth, water, fire, air, and ether (sky).

1) Ether becomes manifested first. Its subtle form is the quality of sound.

2) Because ether is transformed air it generates with the subtle quality of touch. (It also contains the quality of sound.)

3) When air is transformed, fire is generated with its subtle quality of shape or form. (Fire also contains the qualities of sound and touch.)

---

[50] The Orphic Rhapsodies later discarded the figures *Khronos* and *Ananke*, and instead have *Phanes* born directly from *Hydros* and *Gaia*.

[51] *The Alchemy of Voice* p. 20

[52] *Bhāgavata Purana* is one of the "Maha" Puranic texts of Hindu literature, with its primary focus on *bhakti* (devotion). The *Bhāgavata* is widely recognized as the best known and influential of the *Puranas*, and is sometimes referred to as the "Fifth Veda." It is unique in Indian religious literature for its emphasis on the practice of *bhakti*, compared to the more theoretical *bhakti* of the *Bhagavad-gita*; for its redefining of dharma; and for the extent of its description of God in a human form.

4) When fire is transformed, water is generated with its subtle quality of taste. (Water therefore contains the qualities of sound, touch and form.)

5) Finally water is transformed, the element of earth is generated along with its subtle quality of smell. (Earth naturally contains the qualities of sound, touch, form and taste.)

The Relationship between Subtle and Gross Energies

Each of the elements evolve from subtle to gross:
- Sound is the subtle quality of ether
- Touch is the subtle quality of air
- Form is the subtle quality of fire
- Taste is the subtle quality of water
- Smell is the subtle quality of earth

The evolving element naturally has the characteristics of the "parent" element as well as its own. Hence sky, the subtlest of the five gross elements has one only quality, whereas earth, the last element to manifest, has all the qualities of all the elements.[53]

- Ether – sound
- Air – sound, touch
- Fire – sound, touch, form
- Water – sound, touch, form, taste
- Earth – sound, touch, form, taste, smell

Commenting on these relationships, Srila Prabhupada highlights the importance of water:

> The construction of the whole material world is prominently made by three elements, namely earth, water and fire. But the living force is produced by sky, air and water. So water is the common element in both the gross and subtle forms of the material creation. *Water is the*

---

[53] *Srimad Bhagavatam* 3.5.32-36.

59

most prominent element and is therefore the principle element of all the five. [54]

The symbiotic relationship between water and earth is clear – land covers 29.22% of the earth's surface, which is about 57.5 million square miles (149 x 10⁶ square kilometers) and water covers the other 70.78%. This is about 139.4 million square miles (361 x 10⁶ square kilometers) of water.[55] When you look at earth from space, the planet's most prominent feature is its blue-colored water systems.

As a transporter of energy, water has the ability to heal when it is pristine, or to make us sick if it carries bacteria. Nothing is as essential to life as clean water, and yet our supply of clean water is dwindling before our eyes. As water becomes scarcer on our planet, the question must be asked: "Are we failing to hear its message? Is water trying to communicate to us?" said Dr. Masaru Emoto, author of *The Hidden Messages in Water* and *The True Power of Water*. These questions motivated Dr. Emoto's groundbreaking discovery of how water communicates to us.

Energy Associations

Dr. Emoto surmised that if our bodies are made up of mostly water, and if water can be so easily influenced, it follows that the vibrations we expose our bodies to can literally change our lives. The music we listen to, the movies we watch, the environment we live in, and the people we associate with – all affect our physical, mental, and even spiritual health to some degree.

All of these environmental influences are essentially energy vibrations, impacting our physical, mental and spiritual bodies. You have probably experienced that after watching a

---

[54] *Srimad Bhagavatam* 2.10.31 commentary.
[55] Source: Barnes-Svarney, Patricia. *The New York Public Library Science Desk Reference*, p. 372.

particularly violent movie, you came away feeling uneasy or agitated. Conversely, after spending time in the park, among the trees and animals, you feel refreshed and enlivened. There is a stark contrast between the vibrations that each environment emits. Like air, radio, and TV waves, water is also a conduit of influence. Indeed, there has even been scientific speculation over the years about a sort of "water memory."

Water Memory

In the summer of 1988 the science world was rocked by one of the most controversial research papers ever published in the highly respected journal *Nature*. The paper's author, a charismatic French scientist named Jacques Benveniste, introduced the idea that pure water could somehow remember what it had previously contained.

Benveniste started with a substance that caused an allergic reaction, and then diluted it over and over again until there was nothing left except water. He then observed that the pure water still managed to trigger an allergic reaction when it was added to living cells.

If the experiment proved to be valid, it would require the laws of physics and chemistry to be rewritten.

Moreover, the research would have a positive impact on the credibility of homeopathy, because it is a form of alternative medicine that relies on remedies made by diluting the key curative ingredient over and over again until that ingredient has disappeared.

Even Benveniste was shocked by the implications of his own work: "It was like shaking your car keys in the Seine at Paris and then discovering that water taken from the mouth of the river would start your car!"

The Memory of Water is a Reality

Oxford, UK, 01 August 2007 – *A special issue of the journal* Homeopathy, *journal of the Faculty of*

Homeopathy and published by Elsevier, on the "Memory of Water" brings together scientists from around the world for the first time to publish new data, reviews and discuss recent scientific work exploring the idea that water can display memory effects. The concept of memory of water is important to homeopathy because it offers a potential explanation of the mechanism of action of very high dilutions often used in homeopathy.

Therapeutic Waters

The idea that natural waters are therapeutic is accepted throughout most of the world. A case in point is the famous waters of Lourdes in the foothills of the Pyrenees, where apparitions of Our Lady of Lourdes are reported to have occurred in 1858 to Bernadette Soubirous.

Today pilgrims from Europe and other parts of the world gather *en masse* at Our Lady of Lourdes to touch the spring water from the grotto, which is believed by many to possess healing properties.

An estimated 200 million people have visited the shrine since 1860, and the Roman Catholic Church has officially recognized 67 miraculous healings following stringent examination for authenticity. To be deemed authentic, a miracle healing must have no physical or psychological basis other than the healing power of the water.

Water is a Conduit of Intention

Such miraculous powers within water could be explained by the presence of *Undines* (water spirits); however, they could also be the result of focused intention. In other words, so many people want the water of Lourdes to heal that it does just that.

Dr. Masaru Emoto proved that water responds to the intentions and vibrations it is exposed to. "Water is the mirror of the soul," he said, and "it is definitely trying to talk to us." Dr. Emoto believes that water has many faces and that it can align itself with the consciousness of human beings, as his comments in an interview with *Vision Magazine*[56] illustrate:

In the early 90s, I came up with the idea to take water crystal photos and I succeeded using high-speed photography. I discovered that crystals formed in frozen water revealed changes when specific concentrated thoughts were directed toward them. I found that water from clear springs and water that has been exposed to loving words showed brilliant complexity and colorful snowflake patterns. In contrast, polluted water or water exposed to negative thoughts formed incomplete, asymmetrical patterns with dull colors. The implications of this research created a new awareness of how we can positively impact the Earth and our personal health. I have found this experience to be quite mysterious, yet inspiring.

Emoto believes that water is the messenger of God, or a "conduit of Spirit," and that one can improve the quality of their life by "sending healing energy to water." To pray to water, he postulates, is the same as praying to God, because "water is an expression of God."

Emoto's research led him to India, where he took water crystal photos from the holy River Ganges. "The quality of the water was not so good physically," he explained, "yet we could obtain a beautiful shaped water crystal." He speculates that this was probably a result of the multitude of prayers offered from people around the river. Interestingly, in support of Werner Heisenberg's "Uncertainty Principle," he also offered that, had the photographer been Hindu and revered the River Ganges, "then even more beautiful water

---

[56] Excerpt from an interview with Dr. Masaru Emoto by Daphne Carpenter ("The Magical World of Water") *Vision Magazine*, September 2008.

crystals could have been obtained." This, of course, is due to the influence of the observer's vibration.

Emoto discovered that water changes its expression when exposed to particular words and intentions, and that the words "love" and "gratitude" had the most profound impact on the water he tested. He noted that the impact was even greater when the words "apology" and "forgiveness" were spoken with heartfelt sincerity.

When asked if he thought water was in some way conscious, Emoto explained, "...water seems to be receptive to harmonized vibrations and unreceptive to dissonant vibrations....It has the capacity to receive and reflect, inheriting a divine intelligence."

At the 2008 Live H2O Concert for the Living Water Festival, Emoto shared with the audience that water likes music and that "we should sing to it." Many a gardener will attest that plants respond positively to happy music. In fact, in the 1920s Bose[57] demonstrated that plants could "feel pain" and understand affection.

"I am the Taste of Water"

The *Bhagavad-gita*[58] contains a statement from Krishna that illustrates how easily we can raise our awareness of God, just by being conscious while drinking water:

> O son of Kunti [Arjuna], I am the taste of water, the light of the sun and the moon, the syllable Om in the Vedic mantras; I am the sound in ether and ability in man.[59]

---

[57] Sir Jagadish Chandra Bose CSI CIE FRS (1858-1937). Born in a Bengali Hindu Kayasth family, Bose was a polymath: a physicist, biologist, botanist and archaeologist.

[58] *Bhagavad-gita As It Is*, by A.C. Bhaktivedanta Swami, published by Macmillan in 1972.

[59] *Bhagavad-gita As It Is*, Verse 7.8.

The translator, Srila Prabhupada comments: "This is the all-pervasive nature of the Supreme Personality of Godhead. We should mark the important word in this verse from the original Sanskrit: *aham. Aham* means 'person,'" he says.

According to monotheistic traditions within Hinduism, God is both a person and an all-pervading energy. Krishna states later in the *Bhagavad-gita: maya tatam idam sarvam jagad avyakta-murtina*, "By Me, in My unmanifested form, this entire universe is pervaded. All beings are in Me, but I am not in them" (Verse 9.4); or, as French philosopher Voltaire once stated, "God is a circle whose center is everywhere and circumference nowhere." [60]

A practical way to understand this all-pervasive nature of God is through the example of the sun. We understand the constitution of the sun globe by experiencing its all-pervasive heat and light. Although we are 93 million miles away from the sun, we are able to understand what the sun is through its energy, heat and light. Essentially, therefore, the sun and its qualities of heat and light are distinct and yet inseparable.

For example, when the sunshine enters your room, you say, "the sun is in my room." Of course if the sun were really in your room, you wouldn't be around to talk about it. The point is that the sun globe and the sunrays are simultaneously one and different. In the same way, the impersonal, all-pervading energy of the Creator is simultaneously one with and different from the personal features of the Creator. God, the Supreme Person, and God's omniscient energy are essentially the same thing, and yet distinctly different. Such is the inconceivable and apparently contradictory nature of the Supreme.

---

[60] Voltaire (1694–1778).

First Steps in God Realization

The idea that realization of God can be experienced in the mundane act of drinking water is profound to say the least, but certainly believable once we accept the all-pervasive nature of the Supreme. After all, water is just one of the numerous energies that make up this mortal world. Logically, we must conclude: where there is energy there must be an "Energetic" – a source from which that energy flows. That energetic Source, according to the *Vedas* is *Para-Brahman*.[61]

The *Bhagavata Purana* contains a rich description of how we can perceive the presence of God's all-pervading energy or universal form in nature:

> O King, the rivers are the veins of the gigantic body, the trees are the hairs of His body, and the omnipotent air is His breath. The passing ages are His movements... (SB 2.1.33) ...the clouds, which carry water, are the hairs on His head, the terminations of days or nights are His dress, and the supreme cause of material creation is His intelligence. His mind is the moon, the reservoir of all changes. (SB 2.1.34)

Even without these scriptural references, it is easy to perceive the presence of a divine force in our lives, if we only take the time to contemplate. We may argue on specifics of the Divine, but we can all agree on one thing: God in some form or another exists.

The late Mother Teresa encouraged the practice of contemplation as a means to God realization by making it a central component of her mission.

---

[61] *Para-Brahman*: term often used by Vedantic philosophers as to the "attainment of the ultimate goal." There is only one Supreme *Para-Brahman* and all energies and other deities are expansions of this *Para-Brahman*.

"Our life of contemplation shall...gather the whole universe at the very center of our hearts where the Lord of the universe abides, and allow the pure water of divine grace to flow plentifully and unceasingly from the source itself, on the whole of his creation."

In her teachings she urged people to become more thoughtful by taking the time to silence our rushed lives.

"We need to find God, and he cannot be found in noise and restlessness. God is the friend of silence. See how nature - trees, flowers, and grass grow in silence; see the stars, the moon and the sun, how they move in silence ... We need silence to be able to touch souls."

Sometimes, we need to slow down and quiet our mind to be able to appreciate the full value of our current situation. Silence is golden. Author of *The Ragged Edge of Silence: Finding Peace in a Noisy World*, John Francis Ph.D. certainly believes so.

After an oil spill near the Golden Gate Bridge of San Francisco in January of 1971, Francis took a vow of silence, and avoided riding in motorized vehicles for the next 22 years. A strong-willed and opinionated man, Francis decided to see what he could learn from listening and walking wherever he went. In sharing his experience, Francis learned that contemplation is an effective means to enhance our spiritual awareness because it helps us to discover who we really are - and ultimately - to find peace.

Lacking a natural quiet of a previous age, we can accept the benefits of meditation and silence as a way to counteract the anxiety and depression often generated through our association with a noise-polluted world.

Of all the material elements, water is the one that speaks to our body, mind and soul. In its purest form it energizes our body through the process of hydrolysis; as calming tea it can still our mind; as a transporter of higher vibrations it can inspire our soul; and its feminine qualities can embrace and nurture our entire being.

Take the time to fully appreciate this wonderful element and reap the benefits of holistic well-being.

WE ARE LOVED

Unconditionally and without judgment, the material elements of earth, water, fire and air give us light, warmth, breath and sustenance. Unlike your parents and teachers, they have no expectations whatsoever. For example, the air is freely available to everyone, even the most debauched person, day or night. The same is true of Mother Earth. Despite our arrogance and insensitivity, she graciously receives our burdensome energy in the form of waste, and transforms it into something that we can later use to enrich our lives. When we try to connect with her, she always listens and answers. Trees and plants selflessly provide us with oxygen from our recycled carbon dioxide. Water cleanses us physically and energetically without conditions. Every day, without fail, the sun rises to give us light and warmth and to nourish the food we will later eat.

These are practical examples of the love of the Creator and creation itself. The elements are simply the medium of that unconditional love. We should therefore learn to appreciate this unconditional love and reciprocate accordingly. Or what Christian prophecy calls "the time of meeting ourselves again – the coming of a time when love is the language spoken by all."

Nature Meditations

Once we recognize how other living beings are constantly serving us, it becomes perfectly natural to want to respect or serve them. Such a reciprocation of love is the very foundation of any normal relationship. Indeed, in India it is not at all uncommon for a tradesman to worship his tools at the beginning of the day as a show of respect. The tools may appear inanimate, but at a closer look, like us, they too are comprised of the very same natural energies that make up our body. On a microscopic level, life abounds even in the dullest of things.

At the time of creation, the natural elements, namely earth, water, fire, air, and ether, mingle to create the bodies of all manifested entities — the seas, mountains, aquatics, plants, reptiles, birds, beasts, human beings, and demigods. Therefore, we are *all* energetically related.

The understanding that we *are* intimately connected to and dependent upon every living thing in creation can only serve to help us develop the humble frame of mind necessary to evolve spiritually.

So go ahead, hug a tree today, thank the bees, ladybugs, flowers, and even your trade tools for all that they have done for you over the years! Every animate and inanimate object has in some way served you, because all of them have a role to play in the dance of Mother Nature.

As a daily practice, I recommend a simple nature meditation as part of your food yogi evolution. Simply put, it entails connecting with each one of the five core elements: earth, water, fire, air, and ether. Most spiritual traditions do this by way of formal worship. For example, when a priest offers incense in the church they are connecting with the earth element; when purified water is offered, the water element is honored; an oil lamp or candle honors the fire element; flowers represent the element of air; and the most subtle of all material elements, ether, is offered in the form of a ringing bell. Similarly, when using musical instruments we can effectively connect with these five elements: The Indian rattle containing stones is a way to connect with earth; playing a drum helps us to connect with water; the flute or any wind instrument helps us connect with air; cymbals and gongs connect us to fire; and mantra or prayers resonate in ether.

I suggest that in your own individual way, you establish a regular practice of honoring each one of these elements in your life. It need not be part of some formal worship ceremony, but can be easily incorporated into a daily nature meditation. For example, you could connect with the earth element by placing your bare feet on the ground and then honor the importance of the air element by taking deep breaths into your lungs or taking the time to smell a flower; before you splash water on your face or drink water in the morning, take a moment to appreciate the beauty and magic of this most precious element; as the morning sun rises take a moment to glance up and welcome its light and heat into your body, and finally, start a daily practice of including positive affirmations and sacred sounds into your environment. In this way, organize your life so that throughout the day you are consciously aware and respectful of each element.

Sacred Geometry of Whole Foods

Who would have ever thought that an apple could hold the key to the secrets of the universe and our existence?

Vedic mathematician and sacred geometrician, Jain 108 explains: "Our energetic body forms a torus shape; planet Earth is energetically a torus, and a perfect apple is also a torus. All tori are formed by a rotating closed curve and the most classical form is the ring-shaped doughnut."

Jain proposes that the secret to understanding the torus connection begins with the fetus in the womb. "Before any of the limbs have developed, the human form is essentially shaped like a tube torus doughnut, illustrating clearly that the human body is based on the principle of energy in - energy out. The torus is the ultimate geometrical shape - expressing perfection in balance and efficiency," he explains.

Like all spiritual traditions, Jain suggests that complete knowledge can only be obtained by turning inwards to access our core, as illustrated by the turning in of the torus-like apple. "Since ancient times the apple has symbolized the science of immortality, 'Les pomme bleue'. In French the word 'pomme' comes from 'op om,' or sun ball. The word 'apple' also denotes 'eye', 'stone' or anything round. The phrase: 'You are the apple of my eye,' therefore, has deep meaning, suggesting that in the center of our energetic torus is the self (eye)." It is also interesting to note that Adam and Eve were not allowed to eat the "forbidden fruit," suggesting to many sacred geometricians that the ruling Christian elite who compiled the teachings of the Bible did not want the common people to know of the apple's hidden knowledge of our higher self.

Sacred geometrician Don Tolman offers that if we could reduce all the knowledge of our body and the world around us, it would be: "Everything is a tube." Our body and everything in it is basically tube-like. "Sickness is a result of blockages within 'tubes.'" He says. This "tube" concept is just one of the many mysteries revealed within the torus-like apple.

Slicing the apple in half reveals another feature of its mystical nature – the pentagonal arrangement of seeds. Tolman explains that the "pulsating rhythm of living growth follows the pattern of pentagonal symmetry," and is most perfectly expressed in the golden measure or the divine proportion (phi) — a relationship between a small part and a large part of any whole, and mathematically expressed as the ratio of 1 to the irrational number 1.618033... into infinity. In the simplest terms, the small part of a divine proportion is a scale model of the large part, which is a scale model of the whole.

The golden spiral is another aspect of phi's transcendental character and can be seen all throughout nature, including the nautilus shell, ram horn, butterfly wings, tornadoes, whirlpools, ocean waves, spiraled galaxies and in the movements of birds, bees and schools of fish. Thousands of plant species exhibit the golden measure's proportional spacing in the distribution of their seeds and leaves in what is also known as the Fibonacci[62] sequence. Indeed, even the

---

[62] Leonardo of Pisa, famous for introducing Arabic numbers to Europe and discovering the Fibonacci series where numbers unfold by adding the

roots of plants follow the phi ratio of the Fibonacci sequence and most profoundly it can be seen in the distances between the planets within our solar system.

So what does this have to do with health? Well, as it turns out, the human body also perfectly expresses this same divine proportion. "The body begins its existence in the spiral pattern of an embryo and when it has matured the body exhibits the phi proportion in the primary relationship of its parts," explains Tolman.

Indeed, even our DNA resonates to phi. Our DNA is composed of two 3D spirals. Sacred geometrician Stephen Skinner explains that the geometry that governs these spirals can best be seen if you look vertically down them. "What you will see is a structure that is reminiscent of phi, a series of double pentagons that make up the composite axial view of the DNA double coil. Phi is closely related to 'fiveness' and it is integral to the construction of the pentagon (5 sided)," explains Skinner. In other words, the pentacle, which is based on the pentagon, is in perfect phi ratio, and the external torus-shape and internal pentacle arrangement of the "forbidden fruit's" seeds reveal something important about our true nature.

Torus

The Torus is Nature's perfect pattern for evolving life at every scale. This doughnut-shaped energy vortex can be seen everywhere from atoms to galaxies and beyond. Indeed, it appears that the torus is nature's way of creating and sustaining all forms of life. Growing awareness of this amazing pattern is advancing "new energy" technologies and helping scientist to better understand the nature of the "unified field.

---

previous. Natural growth often conforms to the numbers found in this series.

Director of the THRIVE documentary, Foster Gamble says: *"Looking back on almost half a century of research, including thousands of books, films, interviews with experts from diverse fields, if I were to pick one common denominator to all the facets of my quest, it would be the TORUS, the fundamental energy pattern that invites our alignment at every level of our existence for us to survive and thrive."*

The torus is an energy dynamic that looks like a doughnut, wherein the energy flows in through one end, circulates around the center in a perfect Phi spiral and then exits out the other side. This same energy flow can be seen in atoms, cells, seeds, flowers, trees, animals, humans, hurricanes, planets, suns, galaxies and even the cosmos as a whole.

Scientist and philosopher, Arthur Young, explained that a torus is the only energy pattern or dynamic that can sustain itself for it is made out of the same substance as its surroundings – like a tornado.

Each of us is a torus – our bodies covered with a continuous surface or skin like a tube with a hole at both ends (mouth and anus), while, like the Earth, we are also surrounded by our own toroidal electro-magnetic field with energies flowing from North to South-pole and back through the center of the planet.

While each individual's torus is distinct, it is also open and therefore connected to every other torus in a continuous ocean of infinite energy.

Although this torus energy flow is invisible to our naked eye, by scattering iron filings loosely around a magnet you can witness the toroidal shape of this magnetic energy.

It is for these reasons that perfect health is only achieved when we satisfy the bodies yearning for balance, as perfectly expressed in phi ('fiveness'), by eating whole fruits and vegetables that naturally resonate to phi and arranging our lives in such a way that we honor and connect with each one of the **five** material elements (earth, water, fire, air, and ether).

Perfect health therefore can be as simple as embracing **five** key activities:

EARTH

Your diet needs to include a good portion of uncooked whole fruits, vegetables, seeds and nuts. In other words, food in its natural raw state. The modern diet mainly consists of processed foods made from artificial ingredients combined with fruits, vegetable and grains that have been denatured and grown in soils depleted of essential minerals. The result of this is that most people do not get the nourishment their bodies require and therefore feel the need to compensate for this lack of nutrition by spending billions of dollars on vitamin and mineral supplements.

For example, in the production of white flour, up to 84% of the magnesium, 86% of vitamin E, 60% of calcium and 77% of zinc originally present in the grain is lost.

B12

A common problem for vegans and some vegetarians is how to get sufficient levels of B12. For vegetarian, they may be able to supplement B12 through dairy products, however, for the vegan who avoids all dairy, B12 deficiency is a serious issue. Some alternatives to supplements are savory yeast products; however let's consider where B12 comes from in the first place. B12 is a compound of the mineral cobalt, cobalamin, a product of microbes that is ubiquitous around the world. It is a bacterium that lives in well-nourished soils, and especially soils rich in animal manures. Farm animals eat grass and pick up B12 naturally, which is then cultivated in their guts. When people eat the flesh of these animals they get ample B12. However, again, what can the vegan do? How about going straight to the source? B12 deficiency is a modern ailment, simply because of our lives being so disconnected from Mother Earth. If we did, as our ancestors did, and gardened on a daily basis, running our hands through the fertile soil and breathing the beneficial bacteria into our lungs, there would not be any B12 deficiency.

Earthling

It is also important to daily walk on the earth with your bare feet. By connecting directly with the earth, we reset our bioelectrical body through "grounding," just like any electrical system. In a world where most people live in apartments high in the sky and are surrounding by 'oceans' of electromagnetic pollution, it is imperative to take the time to reconnect with Mother Earth on a daily basis.

The late Ota Kte (Luther Standing Bear), Lakota Sioux writer, educator and tribal leader once stated:

> *The old people came literally to love the soil. They sat or reclined on the ground with the feeling of being close to a mothering power. It was good for the skin to touch the Earth, and the old people liked to remove their moccasins and walk with their bare feet on the sacred Earth. The soil was soothing, strengthening, cleansing, and healing*[63]

Steven Sinatra MD, an American integrative cardiologist, believes, "The benefits from the Earth's energy on the brain, heart, muscles, immune systems – and, in turn, the whole body and the aging process – appear to be massive."

WATER

Maintain good hydration by drinking mineral-rich alkaline waters - preferably sourced from a local spring. Start the day of with water and try to maintain a steady hydration throughout the day. Avoid drinking too much when eating. If you cannot drink spring water, at least filter your water. However, keep in mind that tap water, although it might be filtered, is still very much contaminated by its exposure to

---

[63] *Earthling: The Most Important Health Discovery Ever?* (Basic Health Publications, 2010)

negative vibrations, as reported in Dr. Emoto's studies. In other words, it may be physically pure, but energetically, it is still very impure and therefore polluting to our consciousness.

Fluoride

Another thing to be concerned about when selecting your water source is fluoride. Fluoride is actually toxic waste from the aluminum, phosphoric acid and phosphate fertilizer industries. Fluorine has played a significant role in insect control since about 1896 when sodium fluoride and various iron fluorides were patented in England as insecticides.

Millions of tons of fluoride are produced each year. Drinking water is now fluoridated in many countries, including the United States, Canada, New Zealand, Australia, Singapore, Hong Kong, United Kingdom, Ireland, Spain, Turkey, Italy, India and Chile.

According to 48 studies conducted in China and Russia and uncovered by the Fluoride Action Network (FAN), "...fluoride can cause diabetes and osteoarthritis, alter thyroid hormone levels, reduce testosterone levels in males, damage fetal brain, alter behavior in infants, and cause skeletal fluorosis at fluoride levels below 1 ppm (the level added in water fluoridation programs)."

Fluoride is so ubiquitous now that it is present in processed foods made with fluoridated water, fluoride-containing pesticides, bottled teas, fluorinated pharmaceuticals and even teflon pans. FAN believes, "The glut of fluoride sources in the modern diet has created a toxic cocktail, one that has caused a dramatic increase in dental fluorosis (a tooth defect caused by excess fluoride intake) over the past 60 years. The problem with fluoride, therefore, is not that children are receiving too little, but that they are receiving too much."

Pineal Gland

In the 1990s, a British scientist, Jennifer Luke[64], discovered that fluoride accumulates to strikingly high levels in the pineal gland, located between the two hemispheres of the brain. This gland is responsible for the synthesis and secretion of the hormone melatonin, which maintains the body's sleep-wake cycle, regulates the onset of puberty in females, and helps protect the body from cell damage caused by free radicals.

The National Research Council[65] stated that, "fluoride is likely to cause decreased melatonin production and to have other effects on normal pineal function, which in turn could contribute to a variety of effects in humans."

As a calcifying tissue that is exposed to a high volume of blood flow, the pineal gland is a major target for fluoride accumulation in humans. In fact, the calcified parts of the pineal gland contain the highest fluoride concentrations in the human body, higher than either bone or teeth.

In the United States, some evidence[66] indicates that fluoride, via its effect on the pineal, could be a contributing cause to females reaching puberty at an earlier age than in the past.

For centuries there has been much mystery surrounding the full functions of the pineal gland in the human brain. Some ancient civilizations of the world believed the pineal gland was a "gateway" between the spiritual realms and physical reality, suggesting that we, as spirit, incarnate through this gland. The ancient Egyptians believed our

---

[64] Luke J. (2001). *Fluoride deposition in the aged human pineal gland.* Caries Res. 35(2):125-128.

[65] National Research Council. (2006). *Fluoride in Drinking Water: A Scientific Review of EPA's Standards.* National Academies Press, Washington D.C. (NRC, p. 256)

[66] Luke J. (1997). *The Effect of Fluoride on the Physiology of the Pineal Gland.* Ph.D. Thesis. University of Surrey, Guildford.

entrance into matter took place on the forty-ninth day of the embryonic process. Interestingly, it is exactly the forty-ninth day of the embryonic process, that the first pineal gland tissue starts forming.

The pineal gland has often been referred to as the 'third eye' or 'crown chakra' as found in spiritual and religious context. It's shape resembles a tiny pine cone. Ancient Egyptians described the gland as the "Sun" or the "Eye of God," and according to Luke, fluoride should be avoided if one wants to have a healthy pineal gland.

Negative Ions

We all feel a great sense of wellbeing when walking in a forest, by a lake, on the beach, near a waterfall or in fresh snow. Why is this?

It is all because of the existence of negative ions in the atmosphere. Negative ions are electrically charged particles (atoms or molecules) that are present in our body and the surrounding environment. Problems with health and wellbeing arise when there is too many positively charged compared to negatively charged particles. When that happens we feel imbalanced, fuzzy brained and tired.

In our modern life, we are daily bombarded with positive ions from the electromagnetic radiation generated by power lines and household wires, electric heating and air conditioning devices, mobile phones, computers, TVs, microwave ovens, smog, cigarette fumes, synthetic fabrics used in clothing, furniture and house building, or simply a non-aerated space like a stuffy office, car or bus.

These positive ions can damage our cells by changing the acid-alkaline balance in our body, and are believed to be the reason for the deterioration of our physical and emotional well being.

Great water sources to recharge your body with negative ions are:
- Waterfalls
- Morning due present in forests or gardens

- Photosynthesis
- Summer rains
- Sunny weather
- Fresh Snow

According to studies conducted by Bruce Fife[67], the base of a waterfall contains as much as 610 - 3,000 negative ions per cubic inch. Mountains up to 500 ions per cubic inch, the seaside 250, but in a polluted city, negative ions can be as low as 3 per cubic inch.

FIRE

Rising early and gazing directly at the rising sun[68], or at least making sure to get 15–20 minutes of direct sun exposure on our skin on a daily basis is a great way to ensure you are getting enough fire in your body. Sun gazing can also be done at sunset. I discuss more on sun gazing in a later chapter and sun worship in the following pages.

Exposing your forearms to direct sunlight for 15-20 minutes a day is a terrific way to produce Vitamin D. This is particularly important for people living in the far northern or southern hemispheres, where the sun is much lower on the horizon and therefore not as strong.

It is also important to connect with the fire element in other ways. For example, heating your house with a natural wood fire, rather than an electrical system, or cooking your food on actual fire rather than in a microwave oven.

Become aware of the fire element present in your blood, nervous system and digestion. The more you can become conscious of the fire element's important role in maintaining your health and wellbeing, and adjusting your life accordingly, the better off you'll be.

---

[67] *Health Hazards Of Electromagnetic Radiation, 2nd Edition: A Startling Look At The Effects Of Electropollution On Your Health* - by Bruce Fife
[68] Techniques for sun gazing are described later in the book.

AIR

Fresh air is critical to good health. You can increase the aerobic activity of your body quite efficiently, while not stressing your body by practicing yoga or tai chi. Set aside time to do some intense deep breathing to cleanse the lungs of stale air and toxins, while at the same time, invigorating your blood with oxygen. The best time to do this is early in the morning.

A major problem in the modern city lifestyle is the lack of fresh air. Living and working in air-conditioned apartments where air is recycled to reduce electrical bills, and volatile organic compounds (VOCs) are emitted by a wide array of products including paints and lacquers, paint strippers, varnishes, cleaning supplies, air fresheners, pesticides, building materials, and furnishings, causes great stress to our lungs.

These conditions have played a big role in the increase of allergies, respiratory illnesses (such as asthma), heart disease, cancer, and other serious long-term conditions. Some pollutants cause health problems such as sore eyes, burning in the nose and throat, headaches, or fatigue.

Most of us spend too much of our time indoors. The air that we breathe in our homes, schools, and offices puts us at risk for health problems.

My advice: get out everyday to a park or seaside and breathe fresh air into your lungs.

ETHER

Surrounding yourself with positive sound vibration and practicing daily positive affirmations.

In India, the concept of positive affirmation is known as *sankalpa*. Many yoga practitioners use *sankalpa* during their *yoga nidra* (relaxation) sessions. Indeed, it is a long standing tradition in India to use *sankalpa* during meditation or worship in the temple. Before commencing the meditation or worship, the yogi will verbalize their *sankalpa* as a vow in order to empower the intention behind the worship. Once the ceremony is complete, the *sankalpa* is once again stated, thus fixing it firmly in one's consciousness.

To be accurate, *sankalpa* is more of process of formalizing one's intention to achieve a specific goal.

Swami Muktibodhananda, author of *Swara Yoga: The Trantric Science of Brain Breathing,* believes that "*Sankalpa* is the pinnacle of positive thinking and lifestyle. It reflects and innermost desire that is congruent with your belief system about life and where you are heading. Your specifically designed *sankalpa* needs to relate to a feasible goal in your life that enables the expression of your higher self."

It is best to perform positive affirmations or *sankalpa* when the body and mind are in a relaxed state, thus enabling the command to go deep into the subconscious mind.

Controlling what you are implanting into your subconscious mind is one thing, controlling what others are doing to you, is another issue altogether. Therefore, as much as possible, also try to minimize your exposure to the negative vibrations of movies, television and radio.

It is well documented that the emotional content of films and television programs do affect our psychological health. Graham C. L. Davey, Ph.D., a professor of psychology at the University of Sussex, UK believes, "It can do this by directly affecting your mood, and your mood can then affect many aspects of your thinking and behavior. If the TV program generates negative mood experiences (e.g. anxiety, sadness, anger, disgust), then these experiences will affect how you interpret events in your own life, what types of memories you recall, and how much you will worry about events in your own life."

An average American child will witness around 200,000 acts of violence on television by the time they turn 18. This over exposure to violence can make a child less sensitive and increase their tolerance of aggressive behavior since the violence is often portrayed as comedic.

Choose your friends wisely and let them know that you are

on a quest to protect your consciousness from negative input. Remember, you always have a choice, and just like your body, your mind's health is under your direct control.

Sun Worship

The winter solstice occurs exactly when the earth's axial tilt is farthest away from the sun at its maximum of 23° 26'. The seasonal significance of the winter solstice is in the reversal of the gradual lengthening of nights and shortening of days. Depending on the shift of the calendar, the winter solstice occurs on December 21 or 22 each year in the Northern Hemisphere, and June 20 or 21 in the Southern Hemisphere.

Sadly, though, it is a day that most people barely notice, simply because of the distraction of various commercialized holidays. The winter solstice marks the beginning of a new era, a potential blossoming of consciousness and the resurrection of spirit. Astrotheologists say that it marks the day when the Son of God, represented by the actual sun, pauses for three days (dies) before once again ascending (resurrection) in the sky.

Since the event is seen as the reversal of the sun's ebbing presence in the sky, concepts of the rebirth of sun gods are common. In cultures using cyclic calendars based on the solstices, the year is celebrated as reborn and of new beginnings. In Greek mythology, the gods and goddesses met on the winter and summer solstice.

Any way you look at it, it is an auspicious occasion and one that all of us should pay attention to by harnessing the shifting energies to our benefit. We can best do that by offering our respects to the sun with a heart filled with gratitude.

Some Hindus advocate that one need not honor nature directly, but need only to "water the root of the tree" by exclusively worshipping the Supreme Personality of Godhead, the source of all creation. However, a close study of these same devotional traditions reveals that sun eulogy does indeed take place daily in the form of the *Gayatri* mantra. The *Gayatri* mantra, regarded as one of the most sacred of the Hindu hymns, is dedicated to the sun. Hindu priests will privately chant the *Gayatri* mantra three times daily, just before dawn, at noon and finally, at dusk. The sun is also known as *mitra* (friend), affirming the life-giving nature and optimism its light brings to mankind.

The *Mahabharata* describes one of its warrior heroes Karna[69] as being the immaculately conceived son of the righteous Queen Kunti who was impregnated by the sun god. Sri Rama, the hero of the *Ramayana* and husband of Sita is considered the Hindu model of the ideal man. He was the seventh incarnation of Vishnu and is said to have descended from the *Surya* or Sun dynasty.

Srimati Radharani, the divine feminine counterpart of Krishna, and therefore the essence of all forms of the divine Mother, daily worshiped the sun God.

Sun worship was exceptionally prevalent in ancient Egyptian religion. The supreme Egyptian deity, *Ra* was worshiped as the creator of all life, and was typically depicted with a falcon's head bearing the solar disc. From earliest times Ra was associated with the pharaoh. Astrotheologists believe Christianity has roots in sun worship and the references to the "Son of God" are in fact eulogies to the SUN of God.

Modern attitudes towards the sun

In mundane dealings, it is sometimes said that one should not trust a person who doesn't look you in the eye when greeting you. And yet, our hurried lives are causing us to do just that every single day when the sun rises to greet us. We are usually snoring away in ignorance, oblivious to the grace that comes with honoring the sun's presence. The birds and other animals certainly realize the benefits of praising the

---

[69] Karna was a half brother of Arjuna, the great warrior who received the teachings of the *Bhagavad-gita* directly from Krishna.

early morning sun. The early morning is a veritable symphony of song and dance in praise of the sun.

Yogis, brahmanas and *Qigong* practitioners have known of the health benefits of rising early for centuries. In Asian countries, it is common to find thousands of people performing tai chi, meditation, or prayer just before sunrise. The Vedas state that a 48-minute period beginning 1 hour 36 minutes before sunrise, known as *Brahma Muhurta* (Hour of God), is the most powerful time for any kind of prayer or meditation. The Vedic seers claim that this is the time that the cosmic Gods meditate and start to perform their heavenly duties.

Pharmaceutical companies have created paranoia of the sun, which has led to the overuse of sunscreen lotions to protect our bodies from dangerous UV rays. However, it is important to understand that there are some serious dangers associated with sunscreen, starting with the fact that most popular brands contain a large number of toxic chemicals that can actually increase the chances of cancer!

For example, malignant melanoma has been found more frequently in sunscreen users compared to non-users in some studies, states one report[70] and in May 2012, the Environmental Working Group (EWG) agreed, "There's some evidence that sunscreens might increase the risk of the deadliest form of skin cancer for some people," stated the report[71].

The EWG offered three possible explanations:

(1) Sunscreen users tend to stay out longer in the sun and thus expose themselves to more UV radiation than non-users. David Andrews, a senior scientist at EWG, believes it is because, "when using sunscreen, people change their behaviors and feel much more invincible."

---

[70] Westerdahl J, Ingvar C, Mâsbäck A, Olsson H (July 2000). "*Sunscreen use and malignant melanoma.*" Int. J. Cancer.

[71] http://breakingnews.ewg.org/2012sunscreen/

(2) Some chemicals used in sunscreens break down in sunlight and release free radicals, which most scientist believe to be a major component in the development of skin cancer.

(3) Historically many sunscreens have offered little or no protection against UVA rays, which may be what counts most with melanoma.

Similarly, in May 2011, the *Journal of Clinical Oncology* published a report,[72] which found that the areas of the skin that had been treated with sunscreen had non-significantly more melanomas than the untreated controls.

Moreover, the Journal of Photochemistry and Photobiology[73] claimed that some sunscreen ingredients generate reactive oxygen species (ROS) when exposed to UVA, which can increase carbonyl formation in albumin and damage DNA. Most experts agree that DNA alterations are necessary for cancer to occur.

In addition, these "cancer causing" creams block the overall production of Vitamin D in the body. When our bodies are deficient in Vitamin D, either through the overuse of sunscreens or through a lifestyle that keeps us out of the sun's nourishing rays, many negative health consequences occur, including:

- Weakening of the bones;
- Inability to absorb calcium;
- Slowing of cell regeneration;
- Potential for developing various types of cancers;
- Depression.

Also, insufficient sunlight in the short winter days increases the secretion of melatonin in the body, throwing off the circadian[74] rhythm with longer sleep.

---

[72] *Increased Melanoma After Regular Sunscreen Use?*

[73] Elisabetta Damiani, Werner Baschong, Lucedio Greci (2007). *"UV-Filter combinations under UV-A exposure: Concomitant quantification of over-all spectral stability and molecular integrity."*

[74] Recurring naturally on a twenty-four-hour cycle.

Don't be afraid of the light

It seems that not honoring and welcoming the sun into our lives is at the heart of many of our modern day ailments. Most of us get out of bed after the sun has risen, eat some kind of "solar-deficient" processed cereal; commute in sheltered transportation to our office, where we'll work in artificially lit buildings until after the sun has set, only to return home to repeat the pattern. Indeed, modern city life seems to be at odds with our innate urge to live in harmony with nature.

It is time to acknowledge just how beneficial the sun is to our physical, mental, and spiritual health, and seek the early morning light of the sun wherever and whenever you can get it.

Now that we have explored the physical and metaphysical nature of food and the critical importance of the sun and water, it's time to move onto more practical matters - namely, how the food choices we make impact our physical and mental wellbeing, and the environment that nourishes it.

FOOD POLITICS

If people let government decide what foods they eat and what medicines they take, their bodies will soon be in as sorry a state as are the souls of those who live under tyranny.
– Thomas Jefferson[75]

Is Your Food Safe?

Today more than ever, the Federal Government is micromanaging the quality of our food. However, unbeknown to most consumers, they are also passing laws that are dangerous to the public's health and blatantly supportive of big businesses like Monsanto, whose decades-long history of toxic contamination was chronicled in a 2008 *Vanity Fair*[76] article by Donald L. Barlett and James B. Steele. In the article, the authors recount Monsanto's evolutionary journey, from a corporate chemical giant that brought us the infamous chemical weapon Agent Orange[77] followed by the ubiquitous weed killer Roundup®, to finally their claim of being an "agricultural company" dedicated to making the world "a better place for future generations."

The story begins in 1980 with a US Supreme Court decision that extended patent law to cover "a live human-made microorganism" and laid the groundwork for a handful of corporations to take control of the world's food supply.

---

[75] Thomas Jefferson (1762–1826) Third American President (1801 – 09), author of the *Declaration of Independence*.
[76] ©2008 *Vanity Fair*. Excerpt from "Monsanto's Harvest of Fear," by Donald L. Barlett and James B. Steele, May 2008.
[77] Agent Orange is the code name for one of the herbicides and defoliants used by the US military as part of its herbicidal warfare program during the Vietnam war.

Monsanto reacted swiftly to the ruling and, leading the world in genetic modification of seeds, developed seeds to resist its own herbicide, which allowed farmers to spray their fields with Roundup® without killing their crops. The corporation then patented the Roundup Ready® seeds and instigated an aggressive campaign to enforce its patent rights and compel farmers to use its branded products.

The article recounts an astonishing tale of corporate greed, immorality and manipulation, with farmers and consumers as the victims, but here's the bottom line: in little more than a decade, Monsanto's genetically modified seeds have radically altered global agriculture, and today Monsanto is the largest seed company in the world. Monsanto would have us believe that these developments signal progress, when in fact the corporation has seized control of our food supply.

Because articles like this often get lost in the noise and toxic propaganda spewing out from these corporate behemoths' PR departments, most consumers are simply not aware of the damage that companies like Monsanto are inflicting on their health and the environment. To read the article in its entirety, visit:

http://www.vanityfair.com/politics/features/2008/05/monsanto200805

The Business of GMO

Futurist and author of *1984*, George Orwell once predicted: "We may find in the long run that tinned food is a deadlier weapon than the machine-gun." Based on the following information from the *Seeds of Deception* website, run by the Institute of Responsible Technology, Orwell's statement can also be applied to genetically modified food.

A genetically modified organism (GMO) is the result of a laboratory process called genetic engineering (GE) or genetic modification (GM). Unlike crossbreeding or grafting, which produces a new variety of plant or animal by combining the genes of different *kinds* of plants or animals within the same or closely related species, genetic engineering's invasive procedures breach natural barriers and combine the genes of two different *species*.

Genetic engineering may offer potential human health benefits, but the technology is still very crude and the results are unpredictable. If a genetic engineering procedure went wrong, chemical reactions within the cell could be altered, potentially leading to instability, the creation of new toxins or allergens, and depletion in nutritional value. In fact, genetic engineering poses a number of potential health *risks*, from pesticide and antibiotic resistance to unknown effects of consuming new proteins created in the process. Unfortunately, *profits rather than health benefits* have driven the rush to bring GE technology to the market.

The prevalence of genetically modified crops in US commercial agriculture is shocking. The majority of soy, cotton, canola, and corn crops in the US are genetically modified, along with significant amounts of squash, tobacco, and sugar beets. GMOs also find their way to our tables in food products made from these same crops, as well as in meat, eggs, and dairy products from animals that have ingested genetically modified feed. What most consumers are unaware of is that in the US and other countries, laws are in place to exonerate companies from having to state whether their product contains genetically modified ingredients. Which means that if the product does not state: "No GMO" you can pretty much guarantee that it contains ingredients that have been genetically modified.

While there have been virtually no human studies regarding the safety of GMO foods, several studies have found anomalies in animals that ingested GMO feed, including potentially pre-cancerous cell growth; damaged immune systems; smaller brains, livers, and testicles; false pregnancies; and higher death rates.

All over the world, consumer advocates are demanding an end to GM crop cultivation. Despite their cries, however, leaders have done little or nothing to protect consumers from the potential risks.

For more on GMO foods and a list of great resources, visit: www.seedsofdeception.com

The Power of the Plate

The destiny of nations depends on the manner in which they feed themselves. – Jean-Anthelme Brillat-Savarin[78]

Now that you're more aware of the issues surrounding GMO foods, it's time to voice your concern or lead the way by practical action. Start acting according to your conscience rather than your wallet. Ask yourself: is it really worthwhile to save a few dollars buying genetically modified foods when the ultimate purpose of food is to improve health? By purchasing locally grown organic produce, you not only invest in your health but also support a small group of conscious farmers who are standing up and making a positive difference in this world.

By saying no to companies like Monsanto, you are sending a message that you will not be denied the very best for you and your children. You are also sending the message to Mother Nature that you care and respect her for all she has done for you. We simply cannot afford to ignore this matter; we must take positive action to deny the continual exploitation, bullying and diabolical practices of these GMO companies. Our planet and our children are depending on us to initiate change to ensure their future health and wellbeing, and it all begins at our plate.

But what if you can't afford to purchase organic (non-GMO) produce all the time? The good news is that there are some conventional fruits and vegetables that are ok to buy non-organic, based on their level of pesticide residue. These

---

[78] From *The Physiology of Taste* (1825).

92

include asparagus, avocado, cabbage, cauliflower, coconut, kiwi, mango, papaya, peas, pineapple, watermelon, and cantaloupe. Usually anything with a thick skin is somewhat safe.

The Dirty Dozen

Fruits and vegetables are an essential part of any healthy diet, however, many conventional varieties contain extreme amounts of pesticide residue. You might think you can wash this residue off. Wrong. Numerous tests have shown that some fruits and vegetables, even after extensive scrubbing and peeling can still have a pesticide residue. Peeling a fruit or vegetable also strips away many beneficial nutrients.

The good news is that you can reduce your exposure to pesticides by as much as 80% if you avoid the *"Dirty Dozen."* The bad news is that you may have to pay extra money for the organic variety.

The Environmental Working Group (EWG), a 501(c)(3) non-profit organization founded in 1993 uses the power of public information to protect public health and the environment. EWG specializes in providing useful resources like the EWG's *Shopper's Guide to Pesticides*™ to consumers while simultaneously pushing for national policy change. The EWG's *"Dirty Dozen"*[79] list of foods most likely to have high pesticide residues has been regularly updated since 1995.

According to their latest research, apples take the number one spot while kale drops to number 12.

1. Apples

Conventional apples are typically grown using as many as 42 pesticides, including the reproductive toxin Thiabendazole[80].

---

[79] See: http://www.ewg.org/foodnews/summary/.
[80] In tests on animals, high doses of Thiabendazole have caused liver and intestine disorder, as well as reproductive disorders. Effects on humans

Can't find organic? Safer alternatives include watermelon, bananas, and tangerines.

2. Celery

Because celery has no protective skin, it is almost impossible to wash off the more than 60 chemicals used in their production, including Spinosad, that is lethal to honey bees, and Permethrin, a neurotoxin, that according to a study[81] by J.R. Bloomquist et al., 2002, may have links to Parkinson's disease. This is one vegetable you really should buy organic, or choose an alternative for your salad.

3. Strawberries

Because of their delicate nature and closeness to the ground, strawberries are vulnerable to a host of pests and therefore have a long history of pesticide residue. To my knowledge, they have been on this list since 1995. If you buy them out of season, you can be sure that they've been imported from countries that have far less stringent regulations for pesticide use. Up to 59 pesticides have been detected in residue on strawberries, including Captan[82], which has been linked to cancer in the past, and only recently listed as "not likely" by the EPA. If you can't find organic, try substituting with the far safer kiwi fruit.

4. Peaches

These delicate stone fruits are a favorite for lots of pests and so over 60 pesticides are regularly applied to them in conventional orchards, including (in over 30% of cases) the

---

from use as drug includes nausea, vomiting, loss of appetite, diarrhea, dizziness, drowsiness, or headache.

[81] http://www.ncbi.nlm.nih.gov/pubmed/12428726.

[82] **Captan** belongs to the phthalimide class of fungicides and is often added as a component of other pesticide mixtures. It is used to control diseases on a number of fruits and vegetables. It also improves the outward appearance of many fruits, making them brighter and healthier-looking.

neurotoxin Phosmet[83]. Mark Purdey has made the controversial suggestion that Phosmet may have played a key role in the epidemic of bovine spongiform encephalopathy (BSE), otherwise known as "mad cow disease."[84] If you cannot find organic, safer alternatives include tangerines or mangoes.

5. Spinach
First appearing on the list in 2010, conventional spinach has been known to be sprayed with as many as 48 different pesticides, including Permitherin trans, like celery in 50% of plants tested.

6. Nectarines (imported)
As many as 33 different types of pesticides have been found on conventional nectarines imported from overseas, including the neurotoxin Formetanate hydrochloride which is listed as an extremely hazardous substances in Section 302 of the US Emergency Planning and Community Right-to-Know Act[85]. Safer alternatives include papaya and mango.

7. Grapes (imported)
The first thing wrong with conventional grapes is that most are "seedless", and therefore unnatural. The imported varieties present a greater risk to health than those grown domestically. Grapes grown on conventional vineyards can be sprayed with pesticides throughout the entire life cycle and because of the grape's thin skin no amount of washing or peeling will ever completely eliminate this contamination. Some wines can harbor as many as 34 different pesticides.

---

[83] **Phosmet** is on the US Emergency Planning List of Extremely Hazardous Substances. It is highly toxic to bees. See:
http://extoxnet.orst.edu/pips/phosmet.htm
[84]http://www.medical-hypotheses.com/article/S0306-9877(98)90194-3/abstract
[85] (42 USC. 11002). The list can be found as an appendix to 40 C.F.R. 355.

8. Bell peppers

Just like grapes, sweet peppers (capsicums) have thin skins that don't offer much of a barrier to pesticides. Tests have found as many as 49 different pesticides used on the sweet variety of peppers including Methamidophos, classified by WHO as Toxicity Class (1b), or highly hazardous[86].

9. Potatoes

The potato has been on and off the *"Dirty Dozen"* list for years. This popular vegetable can be laced with as many as 37 different pesticides. If you can't find organic varieties, try sweet potato, eggplant, or earthy mushrooms.

10. Blueberries (domestic)

Despite their reputation as a great source of anti-oxidants, blueberries are heavily treated with pesticides (sometimes as many as 52) including small quantities of the neurotoxin Phosmet as well as the hormone disrupter Iprodione. A much safer and healthier alternative is goji berries.

11. Lettuce

Lettuce has been known to have over 50 pesticides including many reproductive toxins like DDE[87], o-Phenylphenol and Diazinon.

12. Kale/Collard Greens

Kale has had a reputation for years as a hardy vegetable that rarely suffers from pests and disease, but in tests in 2010 and

---

[86] Due to its toxicity, the use of pesticides that contain methamidophos is currently being phased out in Brazil.

[87] Dichlorodiphenyldichloroethylene (DDE) is a chemical compound formed by the loss of hydrogen chloride (dehydrohalogenation) from DDT, of which it is one of the more common breakdown products. DDE is fat soluble which tends to build up in the fat of animals. Due to its stability in fat, DDE is rarely excreted from the body, and body levels tend to increase throughout life. The major exception is the excretion of DDE in breast milk, which delivers a substantial portion of the mother's DDE burden to the young animal or child.

again in 2011 it was found to have high amounts of pesticide residue. A safer alternative includes cabbage, asparagus, and broccoli.

Commercial Milk

It is important to understand the distinct difference between traditional milk flowing from protected and loved cows, as opposed to commercial milk that is forcibly extracted from unloved and diseased cows. One is *sattvic* while the other is not.

Ancient Tradition

India is considered the land of the cows; the Vedic tradition is centered on worship of Krishna, the "cowherd boy," and the cow is honored as a "Mother." India is one of the world's oldest civilizations and has existed on cow's milk for tens of thousands of years. Milk is and always will be an integral part of India's culture.

History has proven that cultures can survive for thousands of years and their people live long, healthy lives when there is a symbiotic relationship between humans and animals. Hundreds of millions of Hindus have used *sattvic* dairy products for thousands of years, lending credibility to the notion that dairy products can be safe to consume. To ignore this fact is to allow ourselves to be blinded by our reluctance to even consider evidence that challenges our own personal convictions and the current medical belief.

All Milk is Not The Same

It is important to keep in mind that milk from each different source is unique; that is, cow's milk and human milk are not one and the same. Taken further, the milk that a brown cow produces is different from that of a spotted cow, and within each herd, every individual cow has the ability to produce a unique blend of milk for its calf.

Similarly, even among breast-feeding women, the milk that each woman produces is not exactly the same. By nature's wondrous design, the milk that a mother produces for her child is perfectly suited to that child. Amazingly, even while breast-feeding, a mother's milk can change according to the needs of the child. Obviously, a more subtle influence is present here – the influence of love. In the same way, if a cow is loved and protected, the milk it offers to humans will most certainly be uniquely beneficial. On the other hand, the commercial milk that comes from mistreated and diseased cows is certainly very harmful as is clearly evident from the numerous medical studies on commercial milk consumption[88].

Milk and the Vedas

Although there is substantial support both from the history of India and it's love affair with milk and the Vedic literature, such as the *Ayurveda* about the benefits of consuming *sattvic* dairy, the fact remains that **a large percentage of the current world population are lactose intolerant.**

Lactose intolerance is the inability to metabolize lactose, because of a lack of the required enzyme lactase in the digestive system. It is estimated that 75% of adults worldwide show some decrease in lactase activity during adulthood. The frequency of decreased lactase activity ranges from as little as 5% in northern Europe, up to 71% for Sicily, to more than 90% in some African and Asian countries.

When the *Vedas* were originally spoken this was most probably not the case, and of course there was no such thing as milk contaminated with growth hormones and antibiotics, etc.

---

[88] It is important to note that *all* research on dairy consumption has been conducted on commercial milk only.

Facts About Commercial Milk[89]

Calcium: Green vegetables, such as kale and broccoli, are better than milk as calcium sources.

Fat Content: Based on percentage of calories from fat, butter is 100%, whereas cheddar cheese is on average about 74% and whole milk a whopping 49%.

Iron Deficiency: Milk is a poor source for iron. To get the US Recommended Dietary Allowance of 11 milligrams of iron, an infant would have to drink more than 22 quarts of milk each day. Milk can also cause blood loss from the intestinal tract, depleting the body's iron.

Diabetes: In a study of 142 children with diabetes, 100% had high levels of an antibody to a cow's milk protein. It is believed that these antibodies may destroy the insulin-producing cells of the pancreas.

Contaminants: Conventional milk is frequently contaminated with antibiotics and excess vitamin D. In one study of 42 milk samples tested, only 12% were within the expected range of vitamin D content. Of ten samples of infant formula, seven had more than twice the vitamin D content reported on the label, and one had more than four times the label amount.

Lactose: Three out of four people from around the world, including an estimated 25% of individuals in the US, are unable to digest the milk sugar lactose, which then causes diarrhea and gas. The lactose sugar, when it is digested, releases galactose, a simple sugar that is linked to ovarian cancer and cataracts.

Allergies: Conventional milk is one of the most common causes of food allergy. Often the symptoms are subtle and may not be attributed to milk for some time, if at all, due to milks absurdly favored position on the food pyramid.

---

[89] Source: Physicians Committee for Responsible Medicine. www.PCRM.org

Colic: Proteins from conventional milk can cause colic, a digestive upset that bothers 20% of infants. Milk-drinking mothers can also pass cow's milk proteins to their breast-feeding infants.

Prostate cancer: One of the most common malignancies worldwide, with an estimated 400,000 new cases diagnosed annually. Its incidence and mortality have been associated with [commercial] milk or dairy product consumption in international and interregional correlational studies.[90]

Organic milk

There should be no doubt that it is a huge risk to your health when you consume commercial dairy products. On the other hand, purchasing organic dairy, although a lot safer, *does not* address the issue of lactose intolerance. Neither does it address the fact that the organically fed cows are also sent to slaughter once their milk production drops. This point alone should shake your conscience to the core and make you think twice about supporting these brutal commercial operations. If you insist on making milk a part of your diet, however, there is no better milk than *ahimsa* milk, or pure unhomogenized and unpasteurized milk from cows that are loved, protected are never sent to slaughter. This is the only kind of milk that could be considered *sattvic* or part of a food yogi diet. See: http://www.ahimsamilk.org/

Community Supported Agriculture (CSA)

Never underestimate that a small group of thoughtful, committed people can change the world, indeed it's the only thing that ever has. – Margaret Mead

Community Supported Agriculture (in Canada, Community *Shared* Agriculture), or CSA, is a socio-economic model of

---

[90] Report by Neal D. Barnard, M.D. "Commercial Milk Consumption and Prostate Cancer." (http://www.pcrm.org/search/?cid=157)

agriculture and food distribution in which a community of individuals supports a cooperative farm operation. The farmland becomes the community's farm, with the growers and consumers sharing the risks and benefits of food production. The term CSA is mostly used in the US, but variations on the concept are in use worldwide.

CSA began in the early 1960s in Germany, Switzerland, and Japan as a response to concerns about food safety and the urbanization of agricultural land. In 1984, Jan Vander Tuin brought the concept of CSA to North America, and since that time, community supported farms have been organized throughout the US and Canada. North America now has at least 1,300 CSA farms, with some estimates ranging as high as 3,000.

The CSA System

The typical CSA farm is small, independent, labor-intensive, and family-owned. CSA stakeholders are actually a cohesive group of consumers who fund the farm's budget for a whole season in order to get fresh, wholesome, locally grown foods. CSA is based on the philosophy that the more a farm embraces whole-farm, whole-budget support, the more it can focus on quality and reduce the risk of food waste or financial loss. CSA allows farmers to focus exclusively on growing and therefore helps them to level the playing field in a market that usually favors large-scale, industrialized agriculture over locally grown food. Thus, in CSA, the bond between consumer and producer is exceptionally strong.

CSAs may employ a variety of subscription models to fit their members' budgets, and food may be distributed by pickup or delivery. In any case, the return value of fresh organic produce, grown and picked by people who care about your health and the environment, far outweighs the investment.

CSAs will often work with local "co-op" stores to provide an easy pickup location for members. If there are no CSA's in your community, it's time to start one. Post a notice at your local health food store or go online to find like-minded people to form a CSA group. Then approach your local farmers.

Grow Your Own Food

The best place to seek God is in a garden. You can dig for him there. – George Bernard Shaw[91]

Supporting a CSA operation is certainly one way to access inexpensive, quality food. However, one of life's greatest pleasures is eating freshly picked foods from your own garden. By good fortune, I lived on an organic farm for many years and relished the time I spent carefully selecting fresh vegetables to use in preparing the community lunch.

There is simply nothing better than connecting with Mother Earth by working your hands through the soil – from planting, to nourishing the seedlings, to harvesting the crop. Once you're done, you feel enlivened and fully satisfied. I certainly did, and that happiness translated into the wonderful meals I prepared for my friends and family. It was probably the most natural thing I ever did in my life.

Agriculture is still the world's most widespread occupation and has always been a prerequisite of survival. Half of humankind tills the soil – more than 75% of them by hand. Agriculture is a tradition handed down from generation to generation in blood, sweat, and austerity. During the first half of the twentieth century, household vegetable gardens were a common thing.

And yet, today, many of us by choice or circumstance are artificially removed from this natural experience by large convenience stores and the concrete jungles that make up city and urban life. Rather than plant herbs or vegetables in our yards, most of us keep grass lawns and buy genetically modified "fresh" vegetables that were prematurely harvested

---

[91] *The Adventures of the Black Girl in Her Search for God*, 1932.

months before on slave-labor farms thousands of miles away. After harvest, such produce is transported to cold storage on fossil-fuel powered vehicles, where it is then gassed, frozen or wrapped in plastic and mindlessly stacked on shelves by disgruntled and underpaid laborers.

It is a sad commentary on today that many of us have lost our relationship with food. In most city households, the only relationship children have with food is going to a fast food drive-through, or popping a frozen dinner in the microwave and eating in front of their video game console.

It is relatively easy to grow your own food. In fact there is even a *Dummies* book for it. Many herbs - like basil, coriander, dill, parsley, and chives - as well as vegetables like tomatoes, cucumber, peppers and spinach grow very well in most situations. Sprouting is another easy method of producing nutritious food that can be grown with the most basic equipment like a glass jar, mesh cloth screening and an elastic band and then added to salads and rice. For information about starting a basic herb garden right in your own kitchen, see resources at the end of this book.

We Always Have a Choice

Gardening is something we all should do. It really is the most natural way of reconnecting to our source. As children we loved to play in soil, explore nature and create. Somehow along the way to adulthood we forgot how important that was to us. We disconnected and became a by-product of a society enslaved to television or other forms of distraction. It is such a shame to see the sad and unhealthy faces of Americans eating at places like McDonald's and shopping at grocery stores filled with genetically engineered fruits and vegetables and microwave dinners. No wonder hospitals and the pharmaceutical industry are thriving.

But despite all the artificiality and apparent hopelessness, there is good news in that our individuality and free choice can never be taken away. We *can* change things to improve our situation, even in the most challenging circumstances. Look at the example of world-renowned psychiatrist, Viktor Frankl, author of the classic bestseller, *Man's Search for Meaning*. Dr. Frankl, a Nazi concentration camp survivor, is perhaps best known for practicing and espousing "freedom of will," especially in terms of one's choice of attitude, as a point of departure on the path to meaning. In Dr. Frankl's own words, "Everything can be taken from a man but – the last of the human freedoms – to choose one's attitude in any given set of circumstances, to choose one's way." In other words, in all situations, no matter how desperate your circumstances may appear or actually be you always have the ultimate freedom to choose your attitude. That independence can never be taken away.

Therefore, whenever you confront a situation that is stressful, negative, or somehow challenging, use your free will to list positive things that are or could be associated with (or result from) your circumstance. Expand your imagination and suspend judgment and list whatever comes to mind, no matter how crazy or unrealistic your thoughts may seem at the time. Be free to determine or define what "positive" means to you, and recruit family, friends, colleagues, co-workers, etc., to help you with your list, if necessary. It is an empowering exercise, and I guarantee it will change your entire attitude on life and show you possibilities that you had not noticed before.

Gardening is one way to reconnect to your source and get back to the basics of your unique and individual human existence. A food yogi is a gardener. So start your garden today, even if only in a small way, and see how your entire attitude will change. At the very least you will start to eat more healthily, and that alone can purify your body and clean your mind of the artificial bonds you have allowed to control you.

The Danger of Organic Foods

I knew this heading would get your attention. The truth is, what we consider "organic" and "natural" may not be as we expect.

You see, the current standards for Certified Organic around the world are often so low that organic crops can sometimes be grown using factory-farmed manures and offal that have been proven to contain the very *same toxic products* used in those factory farms. So what is being sold to consumers as "organically grown" is often nothing more than produce grown using the toxic-laden "organic" manure of slaughterhouse animals. People buying "Certified Organic" products and thinking they are avoiding the chemicals that are used in factory farms (and confinement factory-raised animals) are often being horribly fooled.

The claim by these so-called organic farmers is that it is too expensive to produce vegetables without using factory-farmed animal waste. However, the truth of the matter is that there are many "veganic" farmers successfully growing tasty and nutritious produce using only soils and fertilizers from non-violent sources, while avoiding the dangers of antibiotic, hormone and steroid contamination.

If you're worried about chemicals in your food, think twice about buying "Certified Organic" until the standard of what constitutes "organic" is raised; or better yet, take the time to speak with your local farmers about how they produce their crops. Don't fool yourself into thinking that crops grown in toxic-laden, factory-farmed waste aren't going to absorb those same toxins and deposit them in your body. You have the power to change how your vegetables are grown. If you take the time to talk to your local farmers they will listen and change.

When you visit your local farmers' market, ask the farmers how they grow their products. If you are in NY or MA, chances are they apply tens of thousands of pounds of factory-farm waste to their fields every year. Convince them to make a change to a greener (and more importantly, healthier) way of agriculture. Or better yet, start your own garden and subscribe to practices like those listed in *Growing Green* by Chelsea Publishing.

Veganic Agriculture

Veganic agriculture simply means that a farmer uses no slaughterhouse by-products or manures to grow fruits and vegetables, but instead uses green-manure cover crops and plant-based nutrient sources, as well as ground-up rock powders.

Too often, organic vegetable farms (especially the big ones that grow most of the organic produce you buy in grocery stores) rely almost exclusively on slaughterhouse by-products (chicken manure, blood, bone and fish meal) to get nutrients to their plants. According to Ron and Kathryn Khosla of the Huguenot Street Farm[92], a *veganic* farm in New York, "The only commercial sources for these products are factory farms, where animals lead miserable lives and are fed diets of high-pesticide, GMO food riddled with hormones, steroids and antibiotics."

These substances bio-accumulate in the bodies of the animals and in their waste. "To make matters worse," explains the Khoslas, "the packed and unhealthy conditions that factory-farm animals are forced to live in encourages the spread of diseases that may be transferrable to humans. For example, bone meal fed back to cows has been implicated as a possible cause for the spread of mad-cow disease in Europe."

The mere idea of supporting these unscrupulous industries in any way, and particularly by spreading their toxic waste products onto otherwise clean fields, is completely

---

[92] Huguenot Street Farm, 205 Huguenot Street, New Paltz, NY 12561

oppositional to the goal of organic clean living—but it is happening every day, all across the US.

Biodynamic Agriculture

The term Bio-dynamics is derived from the Greek words, *bios* (life) and *dynamos* (energy). It is a system of agriculture that cooperates with nature by recognizing the biological and chemical value of healthy soil. It is a method of farming that respects the land as a living system and focuses on building and maintaining a healthy living soil in order to produce food that nourishes and vitalizes the body and unites the community.

Biodynamic farmers recognize that the earth is a single, self-regulating, multi-dimensional ecosystem and so they seek to manage their farms like self-regulating, bio-diverse ecosystems.

The methods are based on the teachings of Dr. Rudolf Steiner, an Austrian philosopher and scientist. He demonstrated how the health of the soil, plants, humans and animals depends on reconnecting nature with the creative forces of the Universe. Biodynamic methods produce a living soil with dynamic biological activity, in alignment with the rhythms of the sun, moon and planets in the fixed constellations. Steiner believed that by coordinating earthly and cosmic energies, a farmer could create healthy and nutritious plants.

Biodynamic agriculture includes techniques to 'farm the air' as well as the soil, and is the oldest form of organic farming. In addition to normal organic farming practices, such as composting, green manures, and crop rotation, the system uses special preparations based on mineral, plant, and cow manures. These biodynamic "plant elixirs" enhance the bacterial, fungal and mineral processes in the organic farming system.

The biodynamic planting calendar notes the auspicious positions of the sun, moon, and planets for deciding when to apply biodynamic elixirs and liquid cow manures, as well as when to sow seeds, plant, and spray fruit trees and crops.

It should be noted that biodynamic farmers use only manure from cows that lead healthy and natural lives, thus avoiding the toxic manures from factory farms. It is not surprising then that biodynamic farming is very popular in India with more than 500 farms practicing it exclusively.

A modern proponent of biodynamic techniques is Peter Proctor, the New Zealand born farmer and the focus of an award-winning documentary called *One Man, One Cow, One Planet*[93]. In cooperation with ISKCON[94], Proctor and his partner Rachel Pomeroy now teach and work out of the Bhaktivedanta Academy for Sustainable Integrated Living (BASIL)[95] near Mysore.

Food Laws

Food Safety Modernization Act of 2010

Every month, numerous agricultural bills are being pushed into law around the world without public knowledge. One such bill in the US, *The Food Safety Modernization Act of 2010 (H.R. 2751)* was signed into law by President Obama on January 4, 2011. The bill aims to ensure the US food supply is safe by shifting the focus from responding to contamination to preventing it. Sounds harmless? Not exactly.

The Food Safety Modernization Act (FSMA) has given the Food and Drug Administration (FDA) new authorities to regulate the way foods are grown, harvested and processed and the bill appears to be insidiously far reaching. Surprise, surprise, the main backer behind this bill is the chemical giant Monsanto. That alone should ring your alarm bells.

---

[93] http://onemanonecow.com/
[94] ISKCON, The International Society for Krishna Consciousness
[95] http://www.biodynamics.in/ISKCON.htm

Shocked yet? What about the fact that President Obama, appointed Michael Taylor, a former VP and lobbyist for Monsanto, as senior advisor to the commissioner at the FDA. Taylor is the same person who supported allowing genetically modified organisms into the US food supply without undergoing a single test to determine their safety or risks.

Taylor was also in charge of policy for Monsanto's now-discredited GM bovine growth hormone (rBGH), pursuing a policy that milk from rBGH-treated cows did not need to be labeled.

This unholy marriage of food safety and corporate interests is like the "fox watching the henhouse."

H.R. 2751 and other similar food bills[96] have nothing to do with food safety. Their only agenda is giving more control over our dinner tables to the government and self-serving corporations.

However, contrary to numerous reports, the bill does not include backyard gardens. David Plunkett, a senior staff attorney for food safety at the Center for Science in the Public Interest[97] said that backyard gardens were not part of the bill. Plunkett points to a line in Section 105 of the Senate bill that said the rules "shall not apply to produce that is produced by an individual for personal consumption."

It is important to note that large, influential corporations like Monsanto have full-time lobbyists and legal teams working diligently to get similar bills passed that can in some way facilitate their agenda, which, by definition, is to increase the stock value of the company, and not, as their slogan states, "Growth for a better world."

---

[96] To learn more about these bills, visit: http://www.govtrack.us for all US law or the appropriate government website in your country.
[97] http://www.cspinet.org/

Monsanto's Bait and Switch

A few years back Monsanto's slogan was "Imagine™." The absurdity of this marketing is clear—*imagine* a world with vast monocultures of patented, genetically engineered crops producing foods with inbuilt pesticides? *Imagine* the world's staple food crops like wheat, rice, corn and soy being engineered with genes from bacteria and animals and then released into our food chain without a complete understanding of the long-term health impacts? Just imagine!

Despite the claim on the company's home page that it is an agricultural company, Fortune 500 listings clearly state that Monsanto is a top company in the chemicals industry.

Monsanto's vision statement reads as follows:

> *We will deliver high-quality products that are beneficial to our customers and for the environment, through sound and innovative science, thoughtful and effective stewardship, and a commitment to safety and health in everything we do.*

The hypocrisy is so blatant. In the minds of many conscious consumers, Monsanto is the epitome of corporate evil, with its well-documented history of ruthless bullying, corporate greed, and abuse.

One thing for sure, the ruthless pursuit of profit and power, where selfish interest justifies the exploitation of innocent people and other species, is diametrically opposed to a world of peace and prosperity, characterized by universal respect for all living beings and an honoring of their unique role in the drama of life.

Peace and prosperity begins with acting according to Nature's rule of law - that all things are important, and in the grand scheme of things, as spiritually significant as humanity.

Health Comes from Harmony

Happiness is when what you think, what you say, and what you do, are all in harmony. – Mahatma Gandhi

To be healthy is to be in a state of perfect harmony. An example of harmony in nature is when a school of fish move as one unit in order to increase their chance of survival by numbers. It is truly magical to witness this natural phenomena and I cannot help but think that there must be some sort of communication going on among the fish, but what exactly? It appears almost mystical, but is it? Well, it turns out that there is at least some scientific explanation for this behavior.

Large schools of fish swim in complete unison, each darting up and down, back and forth, diving and turning as if their movements are set to music, but this apparent choreographic display is just fish responding to the water movement on their hair-like receptors (similar to those in the human inner ear), called *neuromasts*, which are so sensitive to any change in the water that these fish are able to travel as if connected, in perfect unison.

It is this kind of harmony and interconnectedness that protects and preserves all life. Indeed, it is the most fundamental rule of survival in a complex eco-system, including the great rainforests of the world. Nature has a way of balancing and harmonizing when we leave things in their pure state. Unfortunately, this simple law got lost along the way with the rise of the modern industrial complex, characterized by cutting, burning, changing, denaturing, killing and serving one's self at the expense of everything else.

What the human population needs to understand is that we are actually in the minority and are totally expendable. If irresponsible human behavior doesn't stop soon, nature will once more do what any living organism does when disease is present: expel it.

Al Gore's award-winning documentary *An Inconvenient*

Truth awakened many people to the danger of environmental abuse and the urgent need to change behaviors now, and many responded. Unfortunately, change is not happening fast enough to outpace the changing environment, and scientists are continuously revising their estimates for rising temperatures and sea levels. However, many of the facts presented in the film are now hotly contested, as was evident when in October 2007 a British judge ruled that the movie (*An Inconvenient Truth*) had nine inaccuracies. Shortly thereafter, in reference to this movie, Chris Monckton, wrote "35 Inconvenient Truths," republished with permission by *EcoWorld* that detailed errors in the movie.

Whether Gore's movie has merit or not, what many people fail to realize is that the climactic reactions we see today are the results of abuse from many generations past. In other words, the environmental abuses that are taking place as you read this, with globalization on a rampage and mega-industrial nations like China and India increasing carbon emissions tenfold, will not wreak their full, deadly impact on the planet for many years to come. Again, when there is imbalance, nature has a way of correcting that imbalance in the most efficient manner possible. How? Disease, famine, earthquakes, hurricanes, tsunamis and pestilence, to name just a few.

One startling omission from Gore's documentary was the powerful influence of agro-business (factory farming) on global warming. Not only did Gore not mention the connection but he didn't even hint that consuming less meat could help curb global warming! I wonder if the fact Gore comes from a family of cattle ranchers with intimate ties to the factory farming industry had anything to do with this?

Granted, Gore's documentary did come out before the United Nations FAO report of 2006, which stated that **the livestock sector generates more greenhouse gas emissions as measured in CO2 equivalent – 18% – than transport** and that it is also a major source of land and water degradation.

However, for Gore to exclude animal agriculture as a possible cause for environmental degradation was clearly a calculated decision to pander to corporate sponsors.

Henning Steinfeld, Chief of FAO's Livestock Information and Policy Branch and senior author of the report released the following statement:

> Livestock are one of the most significant contributors to today's most serious environmental problems. Urgent action is required to remedy the situation.

FAO Media Relations correspondent Christopher Mathews commented[98]:

> "With increased prosperity, people are consuming more meat and dairy products every year. Global meat production is projected to more than double from 229 million tones in 1999/2001 to 465 million tones in 2050, while milk output is set to climb from 580 to 1043 million tones.

> "The global livestock sector is growing faster than any other agricultural subsector, providing livelihoods to about 1.3 billion people and contributing about 40% to global agricultural output."

The FAO report[99] also stated that the livestock sector generates 65% of human-related nitrous oxide (from manures), which has 296 times the Global Warming Potential (GWP) of CO_2.

Even more frightening, suggests Matthews, is that livestock production now uses 30% of the earth's entire land surface, mostly permanent pasture. "As forests are cleared to create new pastures, livestock production is a major driver of

---

[98] FAO news room: (November 29, 2006) *Livestock a major threat to environment.*

[99] http://www.fao.org/newsroom/en/news/2006/1000448/

deforestation, especially in Latin America, where, for example, some 70% of former forests in the Amazon have been turned over to grazing".

Probably the greatest environmental disaster created by livestock is the wide scale damage to the earth's increasingly scarce water resources, including pollution, eutrophication, and the degeneration of coral reefs, among other things. "The major polluting agents are animal wastes, antibiotics and hormones, chemicals from tanneries, fertilizers, and the pesticides applied to feed crops," he states.

According to the United Nations (FAO) 2008 report, more than 20 billion cattle, pigs, sheep and goats are slaughtered for food every year in controlled factory farms, and each one of these animals produce waste. **Animal waste is responsible for over 50% of water pollution** in the world, and that includes the great oil spills of recent history.

Let's now move back to the heart of our message, and focus on the very essence of a pure food culture – namely, the search for spiritual awareness. This search begins with the process of negation while simultaneously recognizing the essential nature of this world.

OUR TRUE NATURE

You don't have a soul. You are a Soul. You have a body.
– C.S. Lewis[100]

Solid Matter is an Illusion

The more we break things down, the more we find that everything is just vibrating energy. In fact, the deeper we look into the nature of matter we begin to see that there is *more space* than apparent matter.

For many years quantum physics has effectively removed the naive conception that "seeing is believing." Atoms have revealed themselves to be mostly empty space, while so-called "subatomic particles" are *apparently* waves of energy.

Harvard University physicist P. W. Bridgeman explains:

> *The structure of nature may eventually be such that our processes of thought do not correspond to it sufficiently to permit us to think about it at all...We have reached the limit of the vision of the great pioneers of science.*

Considering these findings, it makes one wonder: what is the true nature of our existence? Am I a physical body? Or does a physical body carry the real "me"? If so, who am I? If this physical body is nothing more than a cluster of vibrating waves of energy, conveniently clothed and decorated by other forms of vibrating energy, then in gross terms, I have been defining myself by the contortions of a skin bag containing decomposing waste matter! Surely, there is more to "me." But what is that something more? Religionists and philosophers

---

[100] Clive Staples Lewis (29 November 1898-22 November 1963), commonly referred to as C. S. Lewis, was an Irish-born British novelist and author of *The Chronicles of Narnia*.

have debated and pondered these questions since the beginning of time.

Bio-chemically, the human body consists of nothing more than oxygen, carbon and hydrogen, with lesser amounts of other chemicals like nitrogen, calcium, phosphorus, sulphur, potassium, etc. If you were to purchase these chemical elements in the same quantities present in a human body, the cost would amount to no more than a few hundred dollars. How did I calculate this? Simply by noting that the majority of the human body consists of oxygen and hydrogen, which is essentially water.[101] Scientists actually state that the average human body is 61.8% water by weight. Protein accounts for 16.6%; fat, 14.9%; and nitrogen, 3.3%. Other elements constitute smaller percentages of body weight.[102] So assuming that 61.8% of our bodies are actually just water, this would mean that an average 150-pound human's water content (92.7 pounds) would be equivalent to 29.23 x (1.5) liter bottles of pure water. Basing this example on a high quality brand like *Fiji* water, which sells for around $2 for a 1.5 liter bottle, the average human body is worth no more than $58.46 in water content. Add to this the protein content (16.6%) or 29.9 pounds, using an average cost of $1.50/40 grams for protein powder we get a total of $282.31. I'll stop there, because I know you get the point, and the remaining major chemical element is carbon, which, along with fat, is pretty much unwanted and therefore of little value. So the average human body is worth (at least in terms of chemical composition) about $340 and change.

So what makes us truly valuable? Well, we now know that it's certainly not the raw chemicals that make up the physical body. The only logical conclusion, therefore, is that there is something more – something intangible to our blunt material

---

[101] http://random-science-tools.com/chemistry/

[102] Source: Rovin, Jeff. Laws of Order, p. 108.

senses ... something that fuels every loving relationship and drives us to interact with our fellow human beings and animals ... something that cannot be measured in dollars and cents ... something transcendental.

Who Are We?

Every man is the builder of a temple, called his body, to the god he worships, after a style purely his own, nor can he get off by hammering marble instead. We are all sculptors and painters, and our material is our own flesh and blood and bones. – Henry David Thoreau

Life is form that endures. It is a form that constantly fights against the restrictions of time; a form that perseveres despite universal laws that drive all organized things towards disorder and chaos. Even more extraordinary, however, is that life is a phenomenon that remains constant, whereas the matter that it communicates through is constantly being renewed. My fingers that speak to you now through these pages have continually renewed their cells since my life began. Every minute of every day, millions of them die and are replaced in my body, and yet I – the "witness" – remain the same, just like a river remains a river even though fresh water runs in its bed. It is a foolish mistake to think that we are simply beings of matter. In truth, we are life forms clothed by matter. We are like living rivers that wind and snake their way through space and time. The real essence of our being continues on, after all matter decomposes.

The French poet Victor Hugo[103] once eloquently stated:

Nothing discernable to the eye of the spirit is more brilliant or obscure than man; nothing is more formidable, complex, mysterious, and infinite. There is a prospect greater than the sea, and it is the sky; there is a prospect greater than the sky, and it is the human soul.

---

[103] Victor Hugo (1802–1885), *Les Miserables.*

117

While the French mystic Teilhard de Chardin[104] offered:

We are not human beings having a spiritual experience.
We are spiritual beings having a human experience.

But how much do we really understand about this simple statement? Do we have a soul, or are we the soul? What is the nature of soul or spirit? Is it eternal? Is it ghost-like? Is it part of the mental plane?

History is filled with opinions on this most sacred of all topics. With simplicity and an air of indifference, the Greek philosopher Epictetus[105] wrote: "You are a little soul carrying around a corpse," while British poet, Lord Byron,[106] although accepting the notion of reincarnation, dared to challenge its utter audacity:

One certainly has a soul; but how it came to allow itself to
be enclosed in a body is more than I can imagine. I only
know if once mine gets out, I'll have a bit of a tussle before
I let it get in again to that of any other.

It is this very thought of being somehow forced to accept another body that unsettles many people and makes them reject the very idea of an identity separate from the physical. Such people, therefore, will prefer to live in ignorance of the soul and, like children that have been denied candy, will reject the concept altogether, much like the "sour grapes" expression offered in Aesop's fable of *The Fox and the Grapes*.[107]

---

[104] French Geologist, Priest, Philosopher and Mystic, 1881–1955.

[105] Epictetus (AD 55–AD 135).

[106] George Gordon Byron, (22 January 1788–19 April 1824), commonly known simply as Lord Byron, was a British poet and a leading figure in Romanticism.

[107] *Sour grapes* is an expression of an unattainable goal and the human reaction to it. More often, it refers to the nature of humans to rationalize why they wouldn't want that unattainable thing anyway. The phrase has come to be synonymous with bitterness in most modern contexts and in

Whether we believe in a soul or spirit or not, we cannot deny the fact that scientists have never been able to create life in the laboratory. There is certainly something missing from a dead body, and so far science has not been able to identify exactly what that is, and most likely never will.

Voltaire[108] stated emphatically that the empirical approach to discovering the soul would never work:

Four thousand volumes of metaphysics will not teach us what the soul is.

However, a former neurosurgeon, Dr. Eben Alexander has plenty to say on this matter in his new book, *Proof of Heaven*. Long before he wrote his book, Dr. Alexander was a life long "science skeptic." He did not believe in consciousness, free-will or the existence of a non-physical spirit, but held firmly to the belief that consciousness was only an illusion created by the biochemical functioning of the brain. But then something happened to him that dramatically turned his worldview upside down.

It all started when e.coli bacteria infected Dr. Alexander's spinal fluid and outer cerebrum. Eventually, the e.coli started eating his brain, resulting in violent fits of seizure, screaming, muscle spasms and eventually a brain-dead coma. During his comatose condition, Dr. Alexander showed no signs of higher brain activity and was kept alive via respirator and IV fluids. Statistically, the death rate for patients with e.coli infections of the brain is 97%, so the attending physicians gave little hope of survival.

But here is the extraordinary thing about this apparent "death sentence." Rather than experiencing darkness during these seven days of unconsciousness, the once hard-core "science skeptic" experienced a vivid and vast expansion of his

---

the materialist age we now live in, there is no shortage of "sour grape syndrome."

[108] Voltaire (1694-1778) was a French philosopher and writer.

consciousness in the afterlife. By the grace of God, Dr. Alexandria was healed of his e.coli infection and restored to normal brain function so that he could attempt to put this experience into words. The full mind-blowing details are described in his book, *Proof of Heaven*.

Dr. Alexander explains that his afterlife experience was so "real" and expansive that the experience of living as a human on Earth seemed like an artificial dream by comparison. He also shares that time is absent in the afterlife; that love is the fabric of existence; all communication is telepathic; that there are multiple universes, and that the sound "OM" was what he heard after his coma.

Spirits in a Material World

According to the *Vedas*, considered the greatest authority on the science of yoga and reincarnation, the entire material creation comprises of eight gross and subtle elements: earth, water, fire, air, ether, mind, intelligence and false ego. Above these energies is the more subtle spiritual energy or *atma* (soul).

The *atma* is covered by these other material elements in the form of a gross body that is determined according to the *atma*'s karma and desire. Until such time that the *atma* is able to transcend the urges and attachments that come with possessing a material body, it must continue in a cycle of repeated birth and death or reincarnation.

The *Gita* states:

> As the embodied soul continuously passes, in this body, from boyhood to youth to old age, the soul similarly passes into another body at death. A self-realized soul is not bewildered by such a change.[109]

---

[109] *Bhagavad-gita As it Is* (Verse 2-13).

A famous student of the *Gita*, Ralph Waldo Emerson[110] once wrote:

> *The soul is an emanation of the Divinity, a part of the soul of the world, a ray from the source of light. It comes from without into the human body, as into a temporary abode, it goes out of it anew; it wanders in ethereal regions, it returns to visit it ... it passes into other habitations, for the soul is immortal.*

> *It is the secret of the world that all things subsist and do not die, but only retire a little from sight and afterwards return again. Nothing is dead; men feign themselves dead, and endure mock funerals ... and there they stand looking out of the window, sound and well, in some strange new disguise.*

According to the *Gita*, it is the presence of the *atma* that makes the physical body animated. Consciousness is the *symptom* of that *atma* or spirit soul. The difference between a dead body and a live body is the presence of *atma*.

> *O son of Bharata, as the sun alone illuminates all this universe, so does the living entity, one within the body, illuminate the entire body by consciousness.[111]*

Walt Whitman[112] once said,

> *I know I am deathless. No doubt I have died myself ten thousand times before. I laugh at what you call dissolution, and I know the amplitude of time.*

---

[110] Ralph Waldo Emerson (May 25, 1803 - April 27, 1882) was an American lecturer, essayist and poet, who led the Transcendentalist movement of the mid-19th century.

[111] *Bhagavad-gita As It Is (Verse 13.34).*

[112] Walt Whitman (May 31, 1819-March 26, 1892) was an American poet, essayist, journalist, and humanist.

The fact is we do not have a single existence. The world that we are most familiar with, the gross physical world, is not the only realm in which you move and react. Every day when you get up, bathe and go to work, you are reverberating on all levels of reality, gross and subtle. Your physical body may walk in the world of matter, but a subtle aspect of you constantly interacts on a level of pure energy. In order to live up to your full potential as a holistic being, you must become aware of the subtle aspect of your nature that is so often ignored in modern society.

Yin Yang

According to traditional Chinese philosophers, the Universe was created out of a force called *wu ji*, which means "limitless nothingness." Out of this infinite force arose two polar forces known as *yin* and *yang*. These *yin* and *yang* forces interact with each other constantly to produce all things. The *yang* world has to do with the physical realm that we wake up to everyday, whereas the *yin* world is the world of energy and spirit. When a person dies, they cross from the *yang* world into the *yin* world. Both worlds are eternal because in essence they are both energetic vibrations. In the grand scheme of things, all energy, whether it is material or spiritual, has a singular Energetic Source. Therefore, what we define as "material" is in fact just a perverted expression of the same spiritual energy. The Chinese have developed a science called *feng shui* to encourage the harmonious interaction between these two realms.

Like us, food, too, has a physical and subtle existence. It reverberates in both the *yin* and *yang* realms and therefore impacts both our physical and subtle bodies accordingly. The art of food selection and combining according to one's unique bodily constitution (as taught in the *Ayurveda*[113]) is an example of how this energy transfer plays out.

---

[113] *Ayurveda* is a system of traditional medicine native to India.

LIFE FORCES

We are the living links in a life force that moves and plays around and through us, binding the deepest soils with the farthest stars. – Alan Chadwick [114]

Qi

For centuries, the great yogis of India and *Qigong*[115] masters of the Orient have known about the amazing power of harnessing and preserving our natural "life-force" or vital energy, otherwise known as *Qi (pronounced: chee)*. To them *Qi* is tied inextricably to breath, life and natural forces. *Qi*, frequently translated as "energy flow," is often compared to Western notions of *energeia* or *élan* (vitalism).

However, today we often see the ideogram for this *Qi* energy written with the component for "rice." Founder of the spiritual path of *Mahikari*, Kotama Okada, believes this association of the word for *Qi* energy to rice "reflects the materialism of our society." He says the ideogram originally represented energy flowing throughout the three realms – the divine, astral, and physical. This is evident because, "the older form of the character was written with the component of 'fire' and not that for rice. Thus, the character for energy originally represented the spiritual energy of God."

Traditional Chinese medicine asserts that the body has natural patterns of *Qi* that circulate in channels called meridians. Symptoms of various illnesses are often believed to

---

[114] American proponent of organic gardening, 1909-1981.

[115] *Qigong* or *Chi kung* is an English form for two Chinese characters: *Qì* (meaning: breathing or energy flow) and *Gōng* (meaning: force or power with the focus upon some result). Combined, the word describes systems and methods of "energy cultivation" and the manipulation of intrinsic energy within living organisms.

be the product of disrupted, blocked, or unbalanced *Qi* movement inside the body's meridians, as well as deficiencies or imbalances of *Qi* in the various organs. Traditional Chinese medicine often seeks to relieve these imbalances by adjusting the circulation of *Qi* (metabolic energy flow) in the body through a variety of therapeutic techniques, which include herbal medicines and teas, special diets, physical exercise (e.g., *qigong, tai chi*), massage, and acupuncture to reroute or balance *Qi*.

Qigong Master, Dr. Yang, Jwing-Ming explains:

> *To understand Qi massage, you must understand that Qi is the bioelectricity circulating in the body. Because it is electricity, it can be conducted or led through electrical correspondence. Actually, everybody has the ability to do Qi healing. To give an example, when people are sad, their Qi is Yin deficient. If you hold their hands or hug them, your Qi will nourish them and they will immediately feel better. We have been doing this instinctively for a long time. The only difference between the average person and a Qigong master is that the latter has trained in Qigong healing, and can therefore be more effective.*

The Electrical Body

Discovery of electricity brought about the promotion of electromagnetic treatments. Over the years many electromagnetic devices, including the "Rife machine" and the most widely marketed "Zapping machine" have been promoted as a means of curing disease. Practitioners of electromagnetic therapy believe imbalances within the energy field of the body disturb the chemical makeup of the body and are therefore the true cause of disease. Although available scientific evidence does not support claims that these alternative electrical devices are effective in diagnosing or treating disease, modern science fully accepts that electrical and magnetic energy exists in the human body. As a result, a number of electromagnetic and electrical technologies have become mainstays of modern medical practice, as the American Cancer Society notes:

> *Electrical energy is used by physicians to restart the heart after heart attacks and is even applied to promote bone growth. Some accepted electrical devices commonly used in hospitals include EEGs[116] to measure electrical activity in the brain and EKGs[117] to measure electrical patterns of heartbeats.*

Vital Energy

This vital electrical energy or *Qi* exists everywhere within and without, including the air we breathe and the food we eat. Its influence on our mental and physical health, as well as the health of the environment, is significant. While we are absorbing this *Qi* energy, we are simultaneously giving off energy, like dust that flies into the air when an object is moved. This "energetic dust" initially resonates with our unique "energetic signature," or psychic fingerprint, and this is why we sometimes continue to "feel" the presence of someone after they have left a place. This "energetic aroma" eventually returns to a more neutral state over time.

The energetic dust we shed from time to time can be charged with our emotions, and it is typically this emotionally charged energy that we feel when we enter a room. This subtle energy comes to us from the sun, the stars, the earth, and every other living thing, because we are all producing *Qi*. This flowing out and absorption of *Qi* characterizes the interdependency of our world – we take in *Qi* from the food we eat, which has been expelled by nature, and in return we expel *Qi* in various ways, to be once again absorbed by nature. However, food need not be straight out of the ground to be

---

[116] Electroencephalogram: record of brain activity.
[117] Electrocardiogram: a record or display of a person's heartbeat.

imbued with *Qi*. The very act of preparing food with loving intention can saturate the food with good *Qi* energy.

Even though it is beneficial to our health to eat food that is high in vital energy, food alone does not contain enough energy to sustain our physical and subtle bodies. We are also sustained by energy produced by the natural environment – typically from the earth, spring waters and the heavens. This connection is so fundamental to our survival that we do it unconsciously. It explains why we feel such a strong urge to visit the ocean or sit among trees. Our bodies absorb raw, universal energy and convert it to a human frequency so our bodies can use it. It's obvious, however, that our bodies require more than the vital energy we obtain through passive means, and thus the esoteric techniques described in the yogic and Taoist traditions can be helpful to fill that gap. Examples of this are the *pranayama*, *breatharian* and sun-gazing techniques, which will be described later.

Prana

Prana is the Sanskrit[118] word for breath, derived from the root *pra*, which means, "to fill," and cognate to the Latin *plenus*, or "full." It is one of the five organs of vitality or sensation, which also include *vac* (speech), *caksus* (sight), *shrotra* (hearing), and *manas* (thought).[119]

In Vedantic philosophy, *prana* is described as the vital, life-sustaining force of living beings, and is therefore comparable to the Chinese notion of *Qi*. In Korean culture, this energy is known as *gi*; Japanese *ki* and Vietnamese *khí*. *Prana* is considered an active principle forming part of any living thing.

---

[118] *Sanskrit*: "refined speech", is a historical Indo-Aryan language and the primary liturgical language of Hinduism, Jainism and Mahāyāna Buddhism. Also known as Deva-Nagari or "Language of the Gods"
[119] *Chandogya Upanisad* 2.7.1.

A central concept in *Ayurveda* and yoga, *prana* is believed to flow through a network of fine subtle channels called *nadis*, similar to the Chinese notion of meridians. Prana's most subtle material form is the breath, but it is also found in blood, and its most concentrated form is found in semen in men and vaginal fluid in women.

According to the *Ayurveda*, the seven structural elements of the body are known as *dhatus*. The *dhatus* are formed from the food we eat. When digested, the usable portion of food becomes *rasa* (lymph), which is the first *dhatu*. From *rasa*, the second *dhatu*, *rakta* (blood) is produced. *Rakta* plus *rasa* combine to produce the third *dhatu*, *mausa* (muscle tissue). This process continues to form the remaining *dhatus*. In order, they are:

Rasa – lymph
Rakta – blood
Mausa – muscle
Medha – fat
Madhya – marrow
Ashti – bone
Shukra – semen (or ovum).

Shukra is also known as *veerya*, or the vital essence. *Veerya* does not remain only in the reproductive organs, but pervades the body and radiates a subtle light known as the bodily aura. With the help of the *sapta-agnis* (heat energies within the body), each *dhatu* converts itself into the next *dhatu*. Therefore, each *dhatu* contains the preceding *dhatus* within itself. *Shukra* (semen) contains all other elements. It follows then that excessive loss of *shukra* through excessive sex will over time destroy all seven *dhatus*.

According to the *Ayurveda*, it would take approximately 60 lbs. of food or four lbs. of blood to replace the *pranic* energy lost in the ejaculation of just 20 cc of semen.

Once a student of Dhanvantari[120], the great teacher of the *Ayurveda* approached his master after finishing his studies and said: "O Bhagavan! Kindly let me know the secret of health now." Dhanvantari replied:

"This Veerya (seminal energy) is verily like Atman (soul). The secret of health lies in the preservation of this vital force. He who wastes this energy cannot have physical, mental, moral and spiritual development."

Whether the person is male or female, if preserved, vital sexual fluids will enrich and strengthen the body, especially the brain, making it fertile to receive enlightenment. It is for this reason that celibacy has been praised throughout history both inside and outside a religious context. Because celibacy is an outer response to an internal dialogue, success can only be achieved through managing the mind. Many top athletes practice short-term celibacy to increase their determination and optimize their physical performance.

Prana was first expounded in the *Upanishads*, where it is part of the worldly, physical realm, sustaining the body and mind. *Prana* saturates all living forms but is not itself the individual soul. In the *Ayurveda*, the sun and sunshine are also held to be a source of *prana*, and metaphorically speaking, *prana* is much like the sunshine that pervades the body as a result of the "sun" or soul within.

In yoga, the three main channels of *prana* are the *Ida*, the *Pingala* and the *Sushumna*. *Ida* relates to the left side of the body, terminating at the left nostril and *pingala* to the right side of the body, terminating at the right nostril. In *pranayama* practices, alternate nostril breathing balances the *prana* that flows within the body. When *prana* enters a period of

---

[120] *Avatar* of Vishnu from the Hindu tradition. He appears in the *Vedas* and *Puranas* as the physician of the gods (*devas*).

uplifted, concentrated activity, the yogic tradition refers to it as *Pranotthana.*[121]

The Five Pranas

In *Ayurveda*, *prana* is further classified into subcategories, referred to as *pranas*. According to the tradition, these are the vital principles of basic energy. In each individual, they make up the subtle faculties that sustain physiological processes. There are five *pranas* or vital currents in the system:

1. *Prana*: Responsible for breathing and heartbeat. *Prana* enters the body through breath and is then transferred to every cell through the circulatory system.

2. *Apana*: Responsible for the elimination of bodily waste through the lungs and excretory systems.

3. *Udana*: Responsible for sounds produced through the vocal apparatus, as in speaking, singing, laughing, and crying. It also represents the conscious energy required to produce these vocal sounds.

4. *Samana*: Responsible for the digestion of food and cell metabolism. *Samana* also includes the heat regulating processes of the body. Auras are projections of this current. Through meditation one can learn to see auras of light around other living entities. Some yogis who do long-term practice on *samana* are able to produce a blazing aura around their body at will. A glowing aura can also be seen in the face of a person that practices celibacy.

5. *Vyana*: Responsible for the expansion and contraction processes of the body, e.g., the voluntary muscular system, including the process of moving food through the digestive tract.

---

[121] Withdrawal of the senses from their sense objects; restraining the mind's outward-flowing tendency.

This leads us to one of the most astonishing traditions coming out of India, that of sustaining oneself by a method of absorbing pure energy directly from the natural world without eating!

Breatharianism

A breatharian is a person who does not eat or drink and is nourished by *pranic* energy. Breatharianism is the claim that food and/or water are not strictly necessary for human nutrition so long as one can absorb sufficient quantities of *pranic* energy.

The claimed ability to subsist without food-based nourishment is technically termed *inedia*. Some breatharians prefer the term "*pranic* nourishment" to breatharianism.

One might wonder why I would include information on this somewhat controversial subject in a book teaching the art and science of spiritual nourishment through food. A closer look at breatharianism, however, reveals that it, too, is centered on the goal of spiritual awakening, albeit through the "digestion" of subtle energy forces.

Breatharianism, however, should not be confused with fasting or dieting, both of which involve minimally sufficient nutrition, or are practiced on an occasional basis. Nor should breatharianism be confused with conditions such as *anorexia nervosa*, in which there is no claim of continued healthy subsistence.

Some sources say that breatharians live off light, some say they live off *prana*, others say it is air. I am certainly not recommending breatharianism as a path to health and longevity, since for 99.99% of the world population it will simply be unattainable. However, fasting from solid food for short periods has proven to be beneficial to health and promotes longevity. In fact, in the *Ayurveda* and in most health traditions, fasting is considered the cure for all disease.

The Science Behind Breatharianism

One explanation of how breatharianism can work is to consider the fact that the body consists of tissues, which in turn are built of chemical molecules that consist of minute atomic structures. Atoms consist of electrons and protons that are built of even smaller elements. As we go deeper and deeper into this micro-universe, we reach a point where matter ceases to exist. Space has often been called the final frontier, but the micro-universe is an equally unknown frontier, since at this level, all we really have is energy, of which the purest form is *prana* or *Qi*.

All matter that exists within the universe, including the human body, is comprised of vibrating energy. The human body is a sophisticated, programmable and simultaneously self-controlled electro-physical-chemical machine with a central management system called the brain. The centers in the brain that manage this energy and chemistry are the pineal and pituitary glands. In this way, the body is maintained and revitalized using these streams of vibrating energy. A breatharian is simply someone who has mastered the art of extracting this pure energy in the most efficient manner possible.

Sun Gazing

Similar to the breatharian is the sun gazer. The system originated with Lord Mahavir of the Jain tradition, who practiced sun gazing over 2600 years ago. Sun gazing has also existed in ancient Egyptian, Greek, and Native American cultures.

Much is not understood about this ancient health practice. However, what is known is that gazing at the sun or exposing our body to high spectrum lighting activates the pineal gland, the glands responsible for the body's circadian rhythm. The pituitary was once considered a "master gland" until it was later discovered that it was actually controlled by the pineal gland. The pineal gland secretes melatonin, which is a powerful antioxidant; controls blood sugar and sleep rhythms, as well as the function of the pituitary gland.

How to Sun Gaze

Considering the dangers associated with looking at the sun, *I do not recommend this practice. You can try it at your own risk.* I have done it successfully and so far my eyes are still healthy and I have experienced an increase in energy and positivity.

To begin the practice of sun gazing it is best to start with a small increment of 10 seconds only and gradually increase by 5-10 seconds every day until you are comfortable and relaxed with the concept of staring at the sun. The key is to be relaxed when you do this and to not hurry the process. Similar to meditating, you need to let go of all thoughts and become immersed in the experience. Your face should be fully relaxed, knees slightly bent and arms at your side.

Initially the rising sun is very bright, but within a few seconds you will start to see it as a beautiful, pure white pulsating orb. Take notice of how your body and mind is responding to this experience as the sun saturates every cell in your body. You may notice an immediate increase in energy and a more positive attitude. Be aware of this healing and completely give your being to the sun. As the minutes of your sun gazing increases over the following weeks, your awareness of your energetic being may heighten dramatically.

It is not necessary to maintain an unblinking stare. Blink as it naturally happens. The key point is to be relaxed. If you find yourself squinting, relax the muscles in your face and eyes. Allow the pure light in. The more open and relaxed the muscles are in your body the more oxygen and energy is able to flow within your cells enabling more light to enter.

The sun is an incredible source of electrical energy. With the aid of sunlight, you can literally recharge every cell and atom in your body to their full capacity.

You may find it helpful to use a watch or ask a friend to

keep tabs on the time. It is important to slowly increase your exposure to the sun so that the rods and cones within your eye can adapt to the increased levels of light. The sun has enormous powers to heal – however, if you choose to try sun gazing, it is imperative to take things slowly.

Naturally, if the sun seems too bright, don't look at it. If you attempt this, be careful, patient, humble and respectful. The sun's rays are less intense when low on the horizon and therefore more tolerable. The UV radiation is naturally lower, so the danger to your eyes is less. Use common sense. If the sun is too bright and feels as though it may be burning your eyes, don't sun gaze.

Man lives on sun gazing

Mr. Hira Ratan Manek was born in 1937 in Bodhavad, India. After retirement, Manek began practicing the ancient system of sun gazing. Amazingly, since the 18th of June 1995, Manek has and continues to live only on sun energy and water! Occasionally, for hospitality and social purposes, he drinks tea, coffee and buttermilk. However, for the last 17 years he has performed three strict fasting sessions, during which time he has sustained himself exclusively on sun energy and water. Independent medical and documentary teams from around the world strictly observed all three sessions.

The first of these fasting sessions lasted for 211 days during 1995-96 in Calicut, India, and was directed by Dr. C. K. Ramachandran, a medical expert on allopathic and Ayurvedic medicine. This was followed by a 411-day fast beginning in 2000 in Ahmedabad, India, and directed by an International team of 21 medical doctors and scientists led by Dr. Sudhir Shah and Dr. K. K. Shah, the President of the Indian Medical Association.

After the reports at Ahmedabad spread, Mr. Manek was invited to Thomas Jefferson University and the University of Pennsylvania in Philadelphia, where he underwent a 130-day observation period. This Science/Medical Team wanted to observe and examine his retina, pineal gland and brain. The observation team was led by Dr. Andrew B. Newberg, a leading authority on the brain who was featured in the movie *What the Bleep Do We Know*, and by Dr. George C. Brenard, the leading authority on the pineal gland. Initial results indicated that the gray cells in Mr. Manek's brain are regenerating. Seven hundred photographs have been taken where the neurons were reported to be active and not dying. Furthermore, the pineal gland was expanding rather than shrinking, which is what typically happens in one's mid-50s, when its maximum average size is about 6 x 6 mm. Mr. Manek's pineal gland, however, was measured at 8 x 11 mm.

The uniqueness of Hira Raten Manek is that he surrendered his body for observation and experimentation by the scientific community for several extended periods. Scientists and doctors acknowledge that hunger is reduced if not eliminated, but due to the complexity of the various brain functions, they have not been able to explain exactly how sun gazing has such positive effects on the human mind or body.

One explanation is that there seems to be a correlation between hemoglobin (in blood) and chlorophyll (in plants). Mason Howe Dwinell[122], a student of Manek, suggests "the effects of the sun on chlorophyll may be related to the effects of the sun on hemoglobin." Hemoglobin has the same chemical formula and function as chlorophyll, except that hemoglobin has iron (Fe) in its center, while chlorophyll has magnesium (Mg). This link between hemoglobin and chlorophyll and the recommended 44 minutes of exposure to the sun to enable all the blood in the body to pass through the retinas[123] is still under research. It is not too farfetched,

---

[122] *The Earth Was Flat*, insight into the ancient practice of sun gazing, by Mason Howe Dwinell. 2005.
[123] The retina is the only place in the body where the sunlight touches the human blood vessels directly or almost directly.

however, to think that the human body, much like a plant, could photosynthesize sunrays into energy that our body can use. Another interesting discovery relating to sun gazing was made in 1979 when Fritz Hollwich showed that light (electromagnetic pulse) entering the eyes helps regulate the autonomic and hormonal processes.

Manek teaches that one should gaze at the sun only during the first hour of sunrise and during the remaining minutes of sunset for small increments of time, gradually increasing the sessions until a maximum exposure of 44 minutes is achieved. At which time, he claims, "one does not have to eat ever again!"

It is important to understand that Mr. Manek achieved his results in a very controlled environment under strict Jain principles. According to Manek, sun gazing is to be practiced standing bare footed on bare earth. You can stand on sand, gravel, stones, mud, or bare soil. Whatever is available. However, standing on tar, concrete, or grass, the results may be a bit slower.

Of course, one glaring shortcoming of the sun gazing path is the abstinence from social eating and the subsequent joy it inspires, particularly when the act is the culmination of devotional ritual or a celebratory event. Even Manek's student, Dwinnel, who although having reached the 44-minute threshold, admitted that he wanted to continue eating with friends and family for the sheer joy of it.

YOGA

What is the purpose of Yoga? The answers to this question run the gamut, from becoming more flexible to achieving full enlightenment. But before we explore those answers, let's first define the word "yoga."

The term "yoga" comes from the Sanskrit root, *Yuj*, which literally means, "to join." In the spiritual sense, it is the process by which the relationship of the individual soul with the Supreme Soul is realized by the Yogi. The soul is brought into conscious communion with the Divine Reality when it is cleansed of all lust, greed, anger, and false ego. Thus, once again made pure, the soul can begin to reawaken its original loving union with God. Essentially, the yoga system is a mechanical way to control the senses and mind and divert their focus from matter to spirit. The preliminary processes are sitting postures, meditation, spiritual contemplation, mastering the air passing within the body, trance, and finally realizing God's presence within.

The *Bhagavad-gita*, undoubtedly the most popular work on yoga, characterizes the yoga student and the yoga master in these words:

> For one who is a neophyte in the eightfold yoga system, work is said to be the means; and for one who has already attained to yoga, cessation of all material activities is said to be the means. (6.3)

> A person is said to be have attained to yoga when, having renounced all material desires, he neither acts for sense gratification nor engages in fruitive activities. (6.4)

> When the yogi, by practice of yoga, disciplines his mental activities and becomes situated in Transcendence – devoid of all material desires – he is said to have attained yoga. (6.18)

The perfected yogi of "steady mind" is described in the *Bhagavad-gita* as follows:

> One who is not disturbed in spite of the threefold miseries, who is not elated when there is happiness, and who is free from attachment, fear and anger, is called a sage of steady mind.[124]

The *Bhagavad-gita* is often referred to as the "Handbook for Humanity." Never in the *Bhagavad-gita* has Sri Krishna restricted the scope of the *Bhagavad-gita* to Hindus or Indians. It is a completely non-sectarian treatise on the science of the soul, meant for anyone inquiring about the purpose of life.

The *Bhagavad-gita* was spoken to guide the soul on the path of spiritual advancement. Sri Krishna's teachings in the *Gita* are presented as principles to his friend Arjuna, who is essentially representative of all other souls. The dominant teaching of the *Bhagavad-gita* is to develop a thorough awareness of God in every aspect of our lives, with Sri Krishna explaining three yoga paths, but then declaring that the single most effective path for enlightenment is *bhakti yoga* or the yoga of devotion.

Yoga paths

The three paths given by Sri Krishna are *karma* yoga, *jnana* yoga and *bhakti* yoga. The first six chapters primarily discuss *karma* yoga, in which the yogi achieves liberation by performing prescribed duties. The last six chapters primarily talk about *jnana* yoga, in which liberation is achieved by worshipping the Lord through one's intelligence. Concealed between these two protective covers, like a pearl in an oyster (the middle six chapters), Krishna reveals the "most confidential of all knowledge," *bhakti* yoga – the path of pure, unconditional loving service. He declares this to be the highest, the easiest and the shortest path to success, and for

---

[124] *Bhagavad-gita As It Is*, Verse (2.56)

one who is fortunate to embark on it, the binding illusions of this material world are dispelled in no time.

The word *yoga* is also applicable in a secondary sense to the numerous practices that are conducive to the final fulfillment of yoga, and as such indirectly lead to final perfection. In other words, though a person in a superconscious state,[125]where the mind and the false ego are completely annihilated may be called a yogi, one who is attempting to achieve perfection in yoga is also called a yogi. Unfortunately, modern so-called yogis and yoga systems are more interested in the physical benefits of yoga. In truth, according to the *Gita*, the main purpose of yoga is learning to forget the illusions of this world. Therefore, a lusty, unregulated and irresponsible person can never become a true yogi.

According to the *Gita*, the highest peace that lies beyond the cessation of material existence is found in reconnecting with the Supreme Personality of Godhead. This is known as *samprajnata samadhi*, in which one's entire consciousness is captured by the personal charm and beauty of God.

Yoga is one of the six systems of Vedic philosophy. Unlike so many other philosophies, this philosophy is wholly practical. Yoga is an exact science based on certain immutable Laws of Nature. Yoga is respected all over the world because it contains the secrets to unlock the realms of peace, bliss, and spiritual satisfaction. Indeed, many great philosophers, mystics and scholars of the West found solace in the science of yoga. There is even speculation that Jesus Christ was a yogi of a superior order. The compiler of the *yoga sutras*[126], Patanjali Maharishi, who lived about one hundred and fifty years before Jesus Christ, was not only a philosopher and a yogi, but a physician as well.

---

[125] A state of complete loving union with God.

[126] *Yoga sutras*: a collection of aphorisms on yoga practice.

The Perfection of Yoga

The highest stage of yoga is a state of absolute peace wherein there is neither bodily attachment nor mundane desire, but complete satisfaction of the soul. Yoga can teach us how to control the flickering nature of the mind and attain liberation. A yogi who attains such a state becomes freed from the cycle of reincarnation, with the concomitant evils of birth, disease, old age and death, and achieves liberation. However, liberation from the bonds of material entanglement is *not* the aim of a true yogi. Bilvamangala Thakura,[127] who in early life had followed the path of impersonalism,[128] but later adopted the devotional path (*bhakti*)[129] of worshipping a personal form of God, explains:

> *If one develops his natural devotional service to the Supreme Personality of Godhead, mukti (liberation) stands before him with folded hands to offer all kinds of service.*

In other words, a bhakti (devotional) yogi is already liberated. There is no need to aspire for different types of liberation. The pure devotee of God automatically achieves liberation, even without desiring it.

The impersonal philosopher believes that spiritual perfection or liberation is attained when the individuality is lost. In other words, everything becomes one, and there is no difference between the knower, the knowable and knowledge. But by careful analysis we can see that this is a false argument.

---

[127] The author of *Sri Krishna Karnamrutham* is Vilvamangalam Swamiyar. (AD 1268–1369)

[128] According to *Advaita Vedanta*, the attainment of liberation coincides with the realization of the unreality of personal self and the simultaneous revelation of an 'Impersonal Truth' as the source of all spiritual and phenomenal existence.

[129] In the Vaisnava traditions, the perfection of liberation is defined as the loving, eternal union with God (*Ishvara*). The *bhakti* yogi attains the abode of the Supreme Lord in a perfected state but maintains his or her individuality, with a spiritual form, personality, tastes, and so on.

Individuality is never lost, even when one thinks that these three principles are merged into one, because the very concept that the three merge into one is another form of knowledge, and since the perceiver of the knowledge still exists, how can one honestly claim that all three have become one? The individual soul who perceives this knowledge still remains an individual. Whether in the material realm or the spiritual dimension the individuality continues; the only difference is in the quality of the identity.

Yoga lifestyle

Equanimity, serenity, and gratitude are all found in yoga. Indeed, anything by which the highest in life can be attained is also a type of yoga. Yoga is thus all-inclusive and universal in its application, leading to all-round perfection of body, mind and soul. Pure food can therefore also be used to achieve success in yoga. In fact, all the yoga traditions of the world demand it, advocating a pure diet of fruits, vegetables and grains. Since equanimity and peacefulness are so essential to yoga, the killing of animals is clearly unjustifiable.

Yoga is primarily a way of life, not something that is divorced from life. Yoga is not inaction, but rather pure action with pure attitude. Yoga is not running away from home and human habitation, but a process of molding one's devotion to home, occupation and society with a new and divinely inspired understanding. Yoga is not renunciation of life, but a spiritualization of life. Controlling the mind and senses is fundamental to all yoga practice. Yoga is never about becoming a human "pretzel," nor is it meant for increasing sexual powers. Yoga's *only* purpose is to reawaken our divine nature and reunite us with God.

Enlightened Karma Yoga

Karma yoga is essentially acting or performing one's *dharma*, or duty, without concern for results or thought of profit – a sort of selfless sacrifice of action to the Supreme. In a more modern interpretation, *Karma* yoga can be viewed as duty-bound deeds performed without allowing the result to affect one's attitude. In the *Bhagavad-gita*, Krishna advocates *Nishkam Karma* (Selfless Action) as the ideal path to realize the Absolute Truth. Performing allocated work without expectations, motive, or thinking about the outcome will purify one's mind and gradually make an individual fit to see the long-term benefits of renouncing the work itself. This enlightened *karma* yoga concept is vividly described in the following verses from the *Gita*:

> You have a right to perform your prescribed duty, but you are not entitled to the fruits of action. Never consider yourself to be the cause of the results of your activities, and never be attached to not doing your duty. (2.47)

> Be steadfast in yoga, O Arjuna. Perform your duty and abandon all attachment to success or failure. Such evenness of mind is called yoga. (2.48)

To achieve true liberation, one must control all mental desires and tendencies to enjoy gross sensual pleasures independent of a thorough understanding of one's spiritual nature. The following verses illustrate this:

> While contemplating the objects of the senses, a person develops attachment for them, and from such attachment lust develops, and from lust anger arises. (2.62)

> From anger, delusion arises, and from delusion bewilderment of memory. When memory is bewildered, intelligence is lost, and when intelligence is lost, one falls down again into the material pool. (2.63)

By raising one's consciousness to the highest level, one can know that everything, including food, has a divine reality. Those who lack such a comprehensive spiritual understanding may try to renounce so-called "material" objects, but although they desire liberation from matter, they are not able to attain the perfect stage of renunciation. Their so-called renunciation is called *phalgu*, or artificial, according to the *Gita*.

On the other hand, a truly enlightened person is aware of the divine essence of all things, and therefore knows how to reconnect everything to its original divine purpose. He does not, therefore, become a victim of materialistic consciousness. For example, to an impersonalist,[130] God is formless energy and therefore cannot eat. Whereas such an impersonalist tries to avoid tasty edibles, a personalist (or *bhakti* yogi) knows that God, being unlimited, is also the Supreme Enjoyer and therefore can eat all that is offered in devotion.

After offering suitable food or preparations to a personal form of God, a devotee accepts the remnants, known as *prasadam*, whereas the impersonalist rejects *prasadam* as material. The *Bhagavad-gita* claims that an impersonalist may rise up to the point of liberation, but because they have not reached a state of absolute satisfaction, they must take birth again.

A Yogi is Regulated

Yoga exists in the world because everything is linked.
– Desikashar[131]

It is true that through the power of mind control we can affect physical reality; however, because we are ultimately a combination of both gross and subtle energy (*yin* and *yang*), it is also true that the mind will follow what the body tells it.

Hence, great yogis will dedicate themselves for years to a regulated practice of eating, sleeping, working, and exercising in order to contain the wayward mind. The *Gita* states:

---

[130] One who does not accept that God has a form.
[131] T.K.V. Desikachar is the son and primary student of Sri Tirumalai Krishnamacharya, a prominent yogi credited with being a driving force behind the resurgence of Hatha yoga in recent decades.

He who is temperate in his habits of eating, sleeping, working and recreation can mitigate all material pains by practicing the yoga system.[132]

In a practical sense, this means that a *food yogi* will control the urges of the mind and senses and establish regular times for eating so that their bodily functions of digestion and bowel movements are optimized. Typically, a healthy person will defecate at least one time a day. However, normal bowel movements vary considerably from person to person. It is the consistency of the stools rather than the frequency that is more important. Your stool should be soft and easy to pass. When you consume a high fiber diet consisting of a lot of fruits and vegetables, and make sure to get your daily allotment of water, your time on the toilet can be as little as 10 seconds! The ideal routine is to train your body so that you defecate immediately after your morning water rehydration therapy. An external shower and then a breakfast of fruits and light grains should follow this "internal shower" and cleansing of the bowels.

Laughter Yoga

Dr. Siddharth Shah from *Greenleaf Integrative Strategies* recently introduced me to the art of laughter yoga. On first look, it seems almost contradictory. We typically look upon yoga as something very serious and meditative, not something to laugh about. But the idea here is to use laughter as a way to connect with the true and natural joy of the spirit within.

The Bible says that when God created the heavens and earth, "The morning stars sang together and all the heavenly beings shouted for joy" (Job 38:7). The psalmist declares, "May the glory of the Lord endure forever; may the Lord rejoice in His works" (Verse 31). Indeed, joy belongs to the very character of God. God is joy. The Bible further states

---

[132] *Bhagavad-gita As It is* (Verse 6.17).

that when God finished creating, He was so elated that He pronounced it, "very good" (Genesis 1:31) and rested or savored His work.

In this sense, laughter or joy can also be a form of yoga. Laughter yoga participants are first encouraged to just relax and give up all inhibitions. The sessions begin with breathing, stretching and relaxing exercises, and then gradually launch into the first of a series of laughter exercises based on a particular theme or scenario. The clear result of these yoga laughter sessions is that one indeed feels happier and more relaxed. The seemingly artificially induced laughter session tricks the mind to respond in the same positive manner it would if the laughter had occurred spontaneously. Matter over mind? Most certainly – and a very good example of how the body sometimes can dictate to the mind.

Ecstatic Modifier

Another example of this phenomenon is what I call the "ecstatic modifier." Simply put, you just use the word "ecstatic" to describe every noun in your sentence or to sum up your feeling. For example: "That last sentence was so ecstatic." Or, "It is really ecstatic just writing about this topic." It is even more ecstatic when you start using the word ecstatic frivolously, as in, "This is an ecstatic laptop that I am using!"

Try it out, and I promise you that very soon you will actually feel ecstatic. It is truly magical and yet a practical example of how the mind will follow what the voice tells it or the body shows it.

Of course, we could apply this same principle to bring about a negative result, or use it to affect the behavior of others, as in the case of neuro-linguistic programming (NLP). NLP is a model of interpersonal communication chiefly concerned with the relationship between successful patterns of behavior and subjective experiences. It is sometimes used as an alternative therapy to educate people in self-awareness and effective communication, and to change their patterns of mental and emotional behavior.

The importance of this concept of our body actions influencing our mind will become more apparent as we discuss the power of the tongue to influence our spiritual awareness. Simply put: what you eat not only affects you physically, but more importantly, it greatly impacts on your mental health and consciousness.

Yoga and Ahimsa

Ayurvedic educator and yoga teacher Scott Blossom believes, "Eating is perhaps the single most important act for one's yoga practice, because nourishment of the body's tissues forms a foundation for nourishment of the mind and emotions."

It is this body, mind, spirit connection that is at the heart of the yoga tradition. What you eat as food influences the quality of your thoughts and consciousness. Food choices are an integral part of the yoga path because according to these same traditions the body is our personal temple. For example, imagine practicing yoga while feeding yourself nothing but meat, white breads, sugar and caffeine. No doubt, your mind and body would be completely disturbed with such a diet. It's easy to see that a balanced, calm mind is much easier to attain if you nourish your body-temple properly. But what exactly does it mean to nourish your body-temple properly? Just how do you eat like a yogi?

Admittedly, taking your yoga practice to the dinner table may be challenging, primarily because the classic yogic texts such as Patanjali's *Yoga Sutra* and the *Bhagavad Gita* don't list any specific foods for following a "yogic diet", but rather talk generally about the alchemical and psychological effect food has when categorized in terms of their principle quality – *sattvic* (goodness), *rajasic* (passion), *tamasic* (ignorance).

Aspiring yogis are warned to be conscious in their choice of foods and encouraged to choose foods from the *sattvic* category, or foods that are fresh, pure, wholesome and pleasing to the heart and mind.

While there is no specific menu for yogis, experts of the tradition agree that a yogic diet should consist of foods that enhance clarity of mind, peacefulness and make the body strong. In other words, a diet that is consistent with the goals of the physical practice.

According to the Ayurvedic tradition, *sattvic* foods include most vegetables, fruits, legumes, whole grains and ghee (clarified butter). In contrast, *tamasic* foods (such as meat, onions and garlic) tend to make the mind dull and the body lethargic, while *rajasic* foods (such as hot peppers, salt and coffee) promote hyperactivity and tend to agitate the mind.

However, it would be naive to suggest that only *sattvic* foods should be consumed. What is best for you and what will best support your yoga practice is also determined by your current physical condition (known in the Ayurvedic tradition as *vikriti*) and your bodily constitution (*prakriti*). Both need to be considered. For example, a person whose physical constitution is low in 'fire' would do well to include more fire foods in their diet, like hot peppers, goji berries and of course more cooked foods, whereas someone with a high 'fire' constitution would do better on a diet of raw fruits and vegetables.

In other words, what you need as an individual may be very different from what someone else needs. Similarly, because your body is constantly changing, what you need now in your life may be very different from what you needed 10 years ago, or will need 10 years from now. The pragmatism here makes you appreciate the wisdom of the ancient sages when they chose not to lay down a strict yogic diet for all to follow, but rather provided guidelines in terms of the spiritual, physical and psychological effects of certain foods on the body, mind and soul.

In the same way that you learn to listen to your body when exercising, you must listen to your body when it comes to food. Only you will know what is right for your body, mind and consciousness. The rules of nutrition and food combining are always overruled by time, place and circumstance, and, more importantly, how each food affects our state of mind and consciousness.

However, despite the unique needs of each body, true yoga

masters will still insist that a yogic diet take into account the core values and philosophical teachings of yoga, specifically the concept of *ahimsa* (or non-violence), which according to Patanjali is the **first rule on the yoga path.** While many modern yoga teachers do teach that *ahimsa* is an important facet of yoga practice, how they put that principle into action varies considerably. Just as different styles of yoga teach different versions of the same poses, yoga teachers will sometimes teach contradictory interpretations of the *Yoga Sutras*. But while personal interpretations are not entirely wrong in principle, it must be understood that **food choices are inextricable from our spiritual evolution,** as clearly stated in the *Bhagavad-gita*[133], the original book on yoga

As Jivamukti Yoga co-founder David Life says, "Not everyone can do a headstand, but everybody eats. Because of this, what you eat has more impact and matters more than whether you can stand on your head".

The interpretation of *ahimsa* is widely debated within the yoga community. David Life, who has been committed to an animal-free diet for decades, actively encourages yogis to see veganism as the only dietary choice that truly honors ahimsa. "In the *Yoga Sutra*, it doesn't say be non-harming to yourself or people who look like you. It just says do no harm," he says.

It is interesting to note that this same kind of loose interpretation of the sacred teachings is also found in Christianity, where the Bible clearly stated, "Thou shalt not kill". There is no room for interpretation here; to "not kill", includes all forms of life and yet modern Christianity does not promote a vegetarian diet, but rather endorses the wholesale killing of millions of innocent animals. Indeed, in many editions of the Bible, the Sixth Commandment has been conveniently changed to: "Thou shalt not murder", thus positioning the argument outside the moral need to respect non-humans.

---

[133] Verses 17.8, 17.9, and 17.10

Clearly, with such varied perspectives, food cultures and personal experiences, developing a diet that reflects your ethics while honoring your physical needs can be challenging. But in the end, most yogis will agree that part of the practice is to at least develop awareness about what you eat and to honor your body and the body of others as a temple of the soul within. Therefore, try and spend time educating yourself about diets you could follow while also learning about the origins and properties of the food you buy. While it's important to listen to your body, it is just as important to explore the parameters of what it truly means to live a life of *ahimsa* and what is important to your spiritual development. .

Yama and Niyama

Patanjali, the compiler of the *Yoga Sutras*, outlines the path to enlightenment through yoga, beginning with the stage of *yama*, or "what not to do." First among these *yama* vows is *ahimsa* (non-violence).

The *yamas* and the *niyamas* of the *Yoga Sutras* directly relate to universal morals and personal observances that should naturally be applied to diet. *Yama* means self-restraint, self-control and discipline. The *yamas* comprise the "shall-not" in our dealings with the external world as the *niyamas* comprise the "shall-do" in our dealings with the inner world. **The very first *yama* is *ahimsa*.**

Ahimsa is abstinence from injury that arises out of love for all, harmlessness, the not causing of pain to any living creature in thought, word or deed at any time. By definition, *ahimsa* suggests that the foods you eat should not cause harm to you or anyone else. The natural questions therefore are: Is the food I am eating causing damage to my body? Was anyone or anything harmed unnecessarily in the creation or processing of this food? If the answer to either of these questions is "yes", you are not practicing *ahimsa* and therefore not practicing yoga in truth.

Ahimsa and principle of *satya* are the two main *yamas*. All other *yamas* are in support of these two. *Satya* means truthfulness in thoughts, words and deeds. Ask yourself, "Am I living a life of integrity?"

The fifth and final *yama* in Patanjali's teachings is *aparigraha*. The term usually means to limit possessions to what is necessary and to not take more than one's allotted quota. A yogi therefore would ask, "Am I eating more than my body needs to be healthy?" Am I wasteful with food? Or, are my eating habits causing others to go hungry?

The Yamas and Meat Eating

No matter how you look at it, taking the life of an animal or supporting the slaughter of an animal simply to satisfy the cravings of your tongue is violent – not only violent to innocent animals, but violent to the earth as well, and therefore a blatant transgression of *ahimsa*. For example, according to Earthsave, every second of every day, one football field of tropical rainforest is destroyed in order to produce 257 hamburgers.

Considering the volume of medical evidence in support of a plant-based diet and the absolutely clear teachings of Patanjali, *Ayurveda* and the *Bhagavad-gita* to avoid foods that are *tamasic* in nature, eating the flesh of animals is clearly damaging to the body, mind and consciousness.

Finally, the principle of *aparigriha* (not hoarding) is also transgressed when meat is consumed by the simple fact that the factory farming of animals is responsible for more than 30 percent of world grain production being fed to animals, rather than humans. Animals like cows and sheep are traditionally grass eaters. The introduction of grains like corn, soy and barley into the diet of factory-farmed animals is a result of ranchers wanting to decrease the time to fatten cattle and increase the yields from dairy cattle.

A vegan way of life (no flesh foods, eggs, dairy, leather or other animal by-products) proactively supports an *ahimsa* lifestyle in the following five ways:

(1) Compassion to animals
(2) Preserving the earth

153

(3) Providing more food for the hungry

(4) Preserving our health

(5) Promoting peace and unity.

Granted, just existing in this world causes some kind of harm to other creatures or the environment. Being vegetarian or vegan, for example, involves taking the life of the plant, which is why some strict practitioners of *ahimsa* like the Jains will avoid root vegetables and only consume fruits, seeds and grains. Eating plants is natural for humans, but because they are much lower on the food chain, less harm is caused. Also, since animals have more developed nervous systems, the pain felt by taking their life is not equal to the pain a carrot feels when you pull it from the ground!

Furthermore, a plant-based diet causes less violence because the animals raised for consumption have eaten tons of grains before they themselves are slaughtered. For example, Steve Boyan, PhD of Earthsave states: "Before a cow is slaughtered, she will eat 25 pounds of corn a day. In her lifetime she will have consumed, in effect, 284 gallons of oil. Today's factory-raised cow is not a solar-powered ["grass-fed"] ruminant but another fossil fuel machine."

If our eating is not based on love and compassion, we are destined to suffer the ramifications of violence. Dr. Gabriel Cousens believes that, "Everything in the universe is food, therefore what we eat is God, and therefore feeds our souls. This awareness that food affects our minds is not owned by yoga alone. The great Greek mathematician and philosopher Pythagoras once said, 'As long as men massacre animals they will kill each other. Indeed, he who sows the seeds of murder and pain cannot reap joy and Love.' "

Cousens also points out that, "Compassion and non-cruelty toward animals are linked morally and spiritually to world peace. Killing an animal for food, even one that we raise ourselves or hunt, is a violent act, which we forget in consuming its flesh."

Even more significant is the fact that when we eat the flesh of these animals, we also ingest the vibration of this cruelty into our consciousness. "The science of Ayurveda also teaches that food is the basis of the physical body, which in turn is the support of the mind. A healthy diet, therefore, is the basis of both physical and mental health and an important foundation for spiritual practice," he contends.

THE TONGUE

Food actually helps you make moral decisions and [have] moral thoughts. It's not just stuff to fill your stomach. It actually gives you a real quality of thought and you realize that this is what the world needs.
– Peter Proctor, Biodynamic Guru

The Most Voracious of All the Senses

If the purpose of yoga is to master the mind and senses, there is no better place to start than with the tongue.

The *Vedas* state that the senses can be "gateways to hell," and the most important and voracious of all the senses is the tongue. It is stated in the *Vedas*, that if one can control the tongue, then there is every possibility of controlling the other senses, including the mind. And with mind control comes true freedom of spirit.

Chanakya[134] once wrote:

My dear child, if you desire to be free from the cycle of birth and death, then abandon the objects of sense gratification as poison. Drink instead the nectar of forbearance, upright conduct, mercy, cleanliness and truth.

So how do we control the tongue? Well, the tongue has two functions: tasting and vibrating, so essentially we are talking about two things we do every day, eating and talking. As mundane as they appear, the truth is, like everything else we do in life, these two activities can be perfected and purified. Therefore, by systematic regulation, the tongue should always be engaged in only tasting the purest of foods

---

[134] Chanakya Pandit (Indian politician, strategist and writer, 350 BC-275 BC).

and vibrating the purest sounds, of which, according to every spiritual tradition, the sound of God's name is paramount. But let's first discuss what the *Gita* says about pure food.

> *If one offers Me with love and devotion a leaf, a flower, fruit or water, I will accept it.* (9.26)

Lecturing on this verse, Srila Prabhupada explains:

> *The process of achieving a permanent state of spiritual bliss is herein described. It can be attempted even by the poorest of the poor, without any kind of qualification. The only qualification required is a heart filled with pure devotion for the Lord. One's material circumstances are not important. The process is so simple that a leaf, water or fruit can be offered to the Lord in genuine love and the Lord will be pleased to accept it. No one, therefore, is barred from the path of bhakti yoga, because it is so easy and universal. Who is such a fool that he does not want to attain the highest life of eternity, bliss and knowledge?*

Another point of interest from this verse is the allusion to a raw, plant-based diet. There are no other foods mentioned here but a leaf, flower or fruit. Commentators on the *Gita*, however, assert that Krishna's declaration suggests all kinds of wholesome vegetarian foods.

Let's look at the original Sanskrit:

patram - leaf; *pushpam* - flower; *phalam* - fruit; *toyam* - water; *yah* - whoever; *me* - unto Me; *bhaktya* - with devotion; *prayacchati* - offers; *tat* - that; *aham* - I; *bhakti-upahritam* - offered in devotion; *asnami* - accept; *prayata-atmanah* - from one in pure consciousness

There is no mention of cooked food, and certainly nothing resembling the remains of dead animals. Rather what is suggested by Krishna is a pure diet of fresh fruits and leafy vegetables in their most pristine form - *au naturel* - naked, just the way nature intended.

In other words, the *Gita* is unequivocally stating that a live plant-based diet is *the* most conducive diet for a yogi. Indeed, many saints of the past subsisted exclusively on a diet of fruits, nuts and seeds. For example, Saint Aibert[135] (1060-1140) ate uncooked foods as part of his religious asceticism, while Leslie Kenton's book, *Raw Energy-Eat Your Way to Radiant Health*, published in 1984, brought attention to the raw food diets of the long-lived Hunza tribes. Then there is the example of *The Clementine Homilies*, a second-century work purportedly based on the teachings of the Apostle Peter, which states:

> The unnatural eating of flesh meats is as polluting as the heathen worship of devils, with its sacrifices and its impure feasts, through participation in it a man becomes a fellow eater with devils.[136]

Clement of Alexandria wrote:

> It is far better to be happy than to have your bodies act as graveyards for animals. Accordingly, the apostle Matthew partook of seeds, nuts and vegetables, without flesh.[137]

The Bible puts it this way:

> Not a word from their mouth can be trusted; their heart is filled with destruction. Their throat is an open grave; with their tongue they speak deceit[138].

Similarly, throughout the Vedic literatures there are descriptions of great yogis who lived in the forests and subsisted exclusively on a diet of wild fruits and cows milk. Indeed, the compiler of the *Vedas*, Vyasadeva, was one such renounced sage. Foraging of wild fruits, flowers and roots is

---

[135] Saint Aibert, or Aybert, of Crespin was a Benedictine monastic and hermit revered for his intense life of prayer, asceticism and devotion to the Rosary.

[136] Homily XII.

[137] The Instructor 2.1; Richard Young, *Is God Vegetarian*, p9.

[138] Psalms 5:9 NIV.

also mentioned as one of the transcendental arts and crafts practiced by the *gopi* Champakalata[139].

Eating a raw, plant-based diet is the oldest food tradition on the planet. The earliest humans ate only raw foods; only after mastering fire did they begin to cook their food before eating it. From the beginnings of recorded history, we find numerous examples of people in countries, like Iran and India, who subsisted on raw, plant-based diets.

In ancient Greece, Pythagoras founded a philosophical and religious school whose inner circle, known as the 'Mathematikoi,' was required to be vegetarian. His most famous student was Hippocrates, the father of medicine and the Hippocratic oath, who stated, "Let food be your medicine." Many believe that Pythagoras and Hippocrates subsisted on a raw, plant-based diet.

Obviously, a raw (uncooked) plant-based diet is not conducive to all climates and all body types; however, the scientific evidence supporting the benefits of a balanced plant-based diet consisting of whole fruits, vegetables, grains, seeds, and nuts is overwhelming.

Australian "Medicine man" and Ayurvedic herbalist, Jay D. Mulder, points out that in classical *Ayurveda*, determining the ideal plant-based diet is not so simple.

"There are two essential qualities of food described, *para* (superior) and *apara* or (inferior). These two qualities are not discussed in Western versions of *Ayurveda*. Understanding these qualities is critical to determining the ideal diet for oneself.

"For example, if you have good *agni* (digestive fire) and the food is prepared in the correct proportions and taken with appropriate digestives like salt and vinegar, during the correct season, and at the right time of day, then a raw food diet would be considered *para* (superior).

---

[139] One of the eight principle maid servants (*gopis*) of Krishna.

"However, if one has weak *agni* or erratic *vata* (air), or slow digestion (*mandagni*) typical of *kapha*, then raw food is generally *apara* (inferior). However, if the raw food is taken in sunny conditions and prepared and seasoned to make it easy to digest then raw food again becomes *para*."

It is absurd, criminal and totally irresponsible for raw food proponents to push an uncooked plant-based food as the *only* diet for all people and all circumstances. Similarly, it is equally unjustified for some Ayurvedic practitioners to assert that food should never be consumed uncooked. The Vedic philosophy of *Achintya bheda abheda tattva* or (inconceivable oneness and difference in all truth) as expressed in the Ayurvedic *para/apara* concept, perfectly places the raw plant-based diet as both superior and inferior based on time, place and circumstance.

Jay Mulder concludes, "The goal of classical *Ayurveda* is *tridosha* or balancing the three faults or *doshas*, and this is non-different from the ultimate ideal of yoga. Food yoga requires us to highlight the ideal of balance and how to convert *apara* to *para*."

The Ingredient of Bhakti

In the Sanskrit verse quoted earlier, the word *bhakti* is mentioned twice in order to declare more emphatically that *bhakti*, or loving devotion, is the only means to approach God. No other accomplishment, such as becoming a learned scholar, renunciant, or great philosopher can induce God to accept some offering of food. Therefore, according to the *Gita*, without the basic principle of *bhakti* (loving devotion), nothing can induce God to agree to accept anything from anyone.

In the *Mahabharata, Santi-parva*,[140] it states: "Whatever acts are consecrated to the Supreme Lord with exclusive single focused devotion, the Supreme Lord Himself accepts them

---

[140] Chapter CLXXI, verse LXIII, written by Vyasadeva.

upon His head." Similarly, *Gita* commentator, Sridhar Swami offers:

> *Even one who has no position in society, who is penniless but clean externally and cleansed internally – if such a being offers the Supreme Lord a fruit, flower, water or even a leaf with devotion in their heart, the Lord will gladly accept and transcendentally enjoy such simple things.*[141]

The Higher Taste

India is the home of not only vegetarian cooking, but also the science of healthful living. The section of the *Vedas* known as the *Ayurveda* is the oldest known work on biology, hygiene, medicine, and nutrition. Sri Bhagavan Dhanvantari, an *avatar* of Vishnu, revealed this branch of the Vedas thousands of years ago. Many instructions of the *Ayurveda* are similar to modern nutritional teachings and are just plain common sense. Other instructions, however, may seem odd, but if given the chance they will prove their worth.

We shouldn't be surprised to see bodily health discussed in ancient spiritual writings. After all, the human body is a divine gift – a unique opportunity for the imprisoned soul to escape the bonds of this material world – and therefore it must be respected. The importance of a healthful spiritual life is also mentioned in the *Bhagavad-gita*:

> *There is no possibility of one's becoming a yogi, O Arjuna, if one eats too much, or eats too little, sleeps too much or does not sleep enough. He who is temperate in his habits of eating, sleeping, working and recreation can mitigate all material pains by practicing the yoga system.*[142]

Balanced and healthful eating has dual importance. Not only does it play an essential role in maintaining bodily

---

[141] Commentary on *Bhagavad-gita*, verse 9.26.
[142] *Bhagavad-gita As It is* (Verses 6.16 and 6-17).

health, but its opposite – overeating, eating in a disturbed or anxious state of mind, or eating unclean foods – is the main cause of *ama* (undigested food), considered "the parent of all diseases," according to the *Ayurveda*.

Proper eating can also help the aspiring transcendentalist attain mastery over his senses. "Of all the senses, the tongue is the most difficult to control," says the *Prasada-Sevaya*, a song composed by Srila Bhaktivinoda Thakura,[143] a prolific author on Vaisnava theology, "but Krishna has kindly given us this nice *prasada* to help us control the tongue," he declares. Thakura thus reveals a mystical quality of food when it is prepared and consumed in a state of devotion.

Lessons from the Ayurveda

Just as our bodies are made up of trillions of independent cells, we, as spirit, are likened to a minute cell in the universal organism. Like our bodily cells, each of us has an individual existence, but none of us is free enough to live independent of the whole. In fact, everything that exists in the external universe has its counterpart in a living being's own personal, internal universe. For example, the flow of nutrients into the body and the outflow of waste from cells also characterize the continuous flow of energies into and out of the bodies of everything within the cosmos, including planets, stars and galaxies.

There is, therefore, no inherent difference between, say, cooking your food in a pot on the stove; "cooking" your food on the stove of your internal digestive "fire," or "cooking a thought" within your mind. In all cases, a form of heat is needed to prepare the physical food or idea for easier assimilation. Flames are used on the external stove; acid and enzymes are used in the digestive tract, and electrical impulses

---

[143] Bhaktivinoda (1838-1914) was among the first Vaisnava scholars to present the teachings of Caitanya Mahaprabhu and the principles of Gaudiya Vaisnava Theology to the English-speaking world.

are used in firing neurotransmitters within the brain, but the principle of cooking is identical.

The *Ayurveda* presents the theory of the Five Great Elements, more properly known as the Five Great States of material existence, to explain how the internal and external forces are linked together.

The following information is based on notes written by Dr. Robert E. Svoboda, a graduate of the Tilak Ayurveda Medical College in Poona, India.

The Five Great Elements

Earth. The most solid condition of the material energy characterized by masculinity, stability, security and inflexibility. Earth is stable substance.

Water. The liquid state of matter characterized by femininity, flux and flexibility. Water is substance without stability.

Fire. The power that can transmute a substance from solid to liquid to gas, and vice versa. Fire's characteristic attribute is action and transformation. Fire is form without substance.

Air. The gaseous state of matter characterized by dynamism, movability and adaptability. Air is existence without form.

Ether. The subtlest expression of matter from which everything is manifested and into which everything returns; the ether or sky is where all events occur.

The Three Doshas

These five elements condense to the three *doshas: Vata, Pitta* and *Kapha*, which are essentially combinations of Air and Ether, Fire and Water and Water, and Earth respectively.

Vata is the principle of active energy in the body. Mainly concerned with the nervous system, *Vata* controls all movements of and within the body.

Pitta controls the body's balance of active and latent energies. All of *Pitta's* processes involve digestion or "cooking," including the "cooking" of ideas in our mind. The enzymatic and endocrine systems are *Pitta's* main field of activity.

Kapha is the principle of latent energy, which controls body stability (Earth) and lubrication (Water). The tissues and wastes of the body that *Vata* moves around are *Kapha*'s domain.

At the cellular level, *Vata* moves nutrients through the blood and expels wastes out of cells. *Pitta* assimilates nutrients to fuel cellular function, while Kapha governs the cell's physical structure.

In the digestive tract, *Vata* is involved in chewing and swallowing food, *Pitta* digests it, so that *Vata* can absorb nutrients and expel wastes, while *Kapha* lubricates and protects the digestive organs.

In the mind, *Vata* is responsible for retrieving previous data from our memory to compare with new data. *Pitta* then processes the new data and draws conclusions, which *Vata* then stores as new memories. *Kapha* provides the stability needed for the mind to grasp a single thought at a time.

Not Substances, but Forces

Kapha is not mucus; it is the force in the body that causes mucus to arise. *Pitta* is not bile; it is the force that causes bile to manifest. *Vata* is not gas, but increased *Vata* causes increased gas. *Vatta*, *Pitta* and *Kapha* are called *Doshas* because the word *Doshas* means "faults" or "things that can easily become imbalanced. When *Vata*, *Pitta* and *Kapha* are out of balance with one another, your bodily system becomes weak and diseased.

Vata, *Pitta* and Kapha are all essential to our survival, but can cause great discomfort if they are allowed to fall out of harmony with one another. This two-faced characteristic exists because as *Doshas*, they are often in error. Their functions are fraught with challenges. *Kapha* must overcome the mutual indifference of Water and Earth. *Pitta* must conquer the natural animosity that Water and Fire feel for one another. *Vata* is forced to use the inert space to try to

165

control the capricious Air. It is therefore surprising that they function as well as they do.

Because they are so reactive, the body cannot tolerate to store the physical manifestations of these *Doshas* for long, any more than a nuclear power plant can afford to store radioactive waste. *Doshas* are therefore eliminated from the body regularly in the course of performing their functions. The force of *Kapha* is continually expelled from the body via mucus, *Pitta* is regularly expelled through acid and bile, and *Vata* is eliminated both as gas and as muscular or nervous energy.

The Six Tastes

How much of each *Dosha* your body produces depends primarily on which tastes you consume. The tastes influence the balance of the *Doshas* in the body. Like the *Doshas*, these six tastes are derived from the five material elements (Earth, Water, Fire, Air, Ether). It is important to understand that these tastes have a profound effect on all parts of the organism, and not merely the tongue.

Sweet. Composed mainly of Earth and Water. Sweet increases *Kapha*, decreases *Pitta* and *Vata*, and is cooling, heavy and oily. It nourishes and exhilarates the body and mind, and relieves hunger and thirst. Sweet produces satisfaction or satiation, which explains why we often like to end our meal with a sweet taste. Overindulgence in sweet taste, however, leads to *Kapha*'s negative aspects, complacency and greed. Complacent *Kapha*, cools the anger of *Pitta* and comforts the fear of *Vata*.

Sour. Composed mainly of Earth and Fire, sour increases *Kapha* and *Pitta*, decreases *Vata*, and is heating, heavy, and oily. Sour refreshes the being, encourages elimination of wastes, lessens spasms and tremors, and improves appetite and digestion. Sour causes evaluation of a thing in order to determine its desirability, which selectively enhances certain appetites. Overindulgence in evaluation leads to envy and jealousy, which may manifest as deprecation of the thing desired, as in the "sour grapes" syndrome. Envious effect increases *Kapha* if envy of another's success incites you to obtain further success for yourself. Otherwise, *Pitta* will increase, as jealousy mutates into anger over the raw deal you feel you are getting from life. Envy helps reduce *Vata* by focusing and heating up your consciousness.

Salty. Composed mainly of Water and Fire. Salty increases *Kapha* and *Pitta*, decreases *Vata*, and is heavy, heating and oily. Salty eliminates wastes, cleanses the body, and increases the digestive capacity and appetite. It softens and loosens the tissues. Salty taste increases zest for life, which enhances all appetites. Overindulgence in zest leads to hedonism, the craving for indulgence in all sensory pleasures physically available to the body.

Pungent. Composed mainly of Fire and Air, Pungent (which is hot and spicy like chili peppers) increases *Pitta* and *Vata*, decreases *Kapha*, and is heating, light and dry. Pungent flushes all types of secretion from the body, reduces all *Kapha*-like tissues (such as semen, milk and fat), and improves the appetite. Excessive consumption of pungent foods can lead to extroversion, over-excitement and cravings for intensity. Over-stimulation leads to irritability, impatience and anger (pungent language or a sharp retort). Pungent taste increases *Pitta* by actively increasing the flow of hormones and digestive juices, making it easier to digest and to manifest anger. It relieves *Kapha* by decreasing self-satisfaction, and temporarily relieves *Vata* by permitting expression of bottled-up resentment. In the long run, however, Pungent increases *Vata* by exhausting the organs and glands, leading to dryness and an inability to project emotions.

Bitter. Composed mainly of Air and Space, Bitter increases *Vata*, decreases *Pitta* and *Kapha*, and is cooling, light and dry. Bitter purifies and dries all secretions, is anti-aphrodisiac, and tones the organism by returning all tastes to normal balance. It increases appetite, controls skin diseases and fevers, and produces dissatisfaction, which creates a desire to change. When you have to swallow a "bitter pill," its bitterness dispels your self-delusion and forces you to face reality. Too much disappointment leads to frustration, which confirms your system in bitterness. Grief is also bitter. Bitter, however, is the best of all six tastes. As Dr. Vasant Lad explains, "Bitter is better." In small amounts, Bitter helps balance all other tastes in the body. Just as mild dissatisfaction with yourself or your situation impels you to change, Bitter dilates channels which are too constricted, thus reducing *Kapha* and its complacency, and constricts those which are over dilated, thus reducing *Pitta* and its anger. Overuse of Bitter increases *Vata,* as dissatisfaction and continuous change induces insecurity and fear.

Astringent. Composed mainly of Air and Earth, Astringent (which makes your mouth pucker) increases *Vata,* decreases *Pitta* and *Kapha,* and is cooling, light and dry. Astringent heals, purifies and constricts all parts of the body. It reduces all secretions, is anti-aphrodisiac, and produces introversion, the tendency away from excitement and stimulation. Excessive introversion leads to insecurity, anxiety and fear. Astringency causes contraction, which makes you "shrivel like a prune" and clamps the "cold, bony hand of fear" around your throat. Astringent taste constricts, drawing one away from the self-satisfaction of *Kapha* and the self-aggrandizement of *Pitta*. Its constriction increases fear of insufficient sensory "nutrition" and leads to increased *Vata*.

All six tastes are essential for proper functioning of the body, and they all reach us primarily through food.

Your Personal Constitution

Your personal constitution, which is your individual metabolic makeup, helps determine how much effect specific tastes and emotions have on you. This is why everyone who eats the same food does not experience exactly the same mental and physical effects from it. When all the members of a family enjoy a meal together, each individual's tastes and emotions will be affected according to their own individual taste and emotional balance.

Your inborn metabolic pattern is called *Prakrti*, which also means Nature. Your constitution is that set of metabolic tendencies which determine how your body and mind will instinctively react when they are confronted by a stimulus.

Knowing your constitution allows you to know your body and mind better. With this understanding, there is no need to feel guilty for dietary preferences, or for mental traits like anger or fear. Once you understand that these traits are primarily determined by your constitution, lifestyle changes can help your organism minimize their influence. You can get a good understanding of your *Dosha* constitution by a simple analysis of your bodily characteristics, all of which are described in *Ayurvedic* literature.

Your Constitution also Influences your Emotions.

Your personal constitution was determined by the state of the bodies of your mother and father at the time of your conception. That certain sperm which could best endure the conditions prevalent in those two bodies won the race to reach the ovum, and its genes mingled with the genes in the ovum to form the new child.

Your constitution is influenced by your parent's genetics, by your mother's diet and habits during her pregnancy, and by events at the time of your birth. Once your personal constitution and its accompanying tendencies have been set, they cannot be permanently altered. Like your genes, you have your constitution for the rest of your life, like it or not.

You can, however, learn to adjust for your constitution so that you are less affected by its distortions. You can learn how to prevent health imbalances and how to best treat them when they arise. You can know the prognosis of any disease you might contract, and you can determine which rejuvenation program will be best for you. Through study and use of Ayurvedic principles, you can also understand why your spouse, children, relatives, friends, neighbors and co-workers do the things they do, and determine how best to interact with them for maximum interpersonal harmony. You can plan meals for your family according to what is best for each of their *prakrtis*. The bottom line is: through knowledge of *Ayurveda*, you can improve the quality of your life and the life of others through proper food choices.

Because every individual is composed of a body, a mind and a spirit, the ancient *Rishis* of India organized their wisdom into three bodies of knowledge: *Ayurveda*, which deals mainly with the physical body; *yoga*, which deals mainly with the spirit; and *tantra*, which is mainly concerned with the mind. The philosophy of all three are complementary; only their manifestations differ because of differing emphasis.

The Power of Words

In the beginning was the Word, and the Word was with God, and the Word was God. – John 1:1

The other function of the tongue is to vibrate. All humans understand the power of the spoken word. Its sonic energy can be harnessed to inspire, to manifest, to heal and to manipulate the subtle and physical worlds. Both the original Hebrew and Sanskrit alphabets, considered to be given by the gods, state that acts of creation begin in sound. Thus, the Bible states: "In the beginning was Logo [Word]," whereas the *Vedas* claim that the great Architect, Lord Brahma, was inspired by the *Gayatri-mantra* to create this material universe. The *Gautamiya-tantra* states: "From the syllable *klim* (in the *Gayatri* mantra), the universe was created. This syllable is thus the very life and the principal sound of the *srutis* (*Upaniṇads* and *Vedas*). From the letter *l*, earth arose; from the *k*, water arose; from the *i*, fire arose; from the *m*, air arose; and from the bindu (dot above the *m*), ether arose. Thus the mantra is composed of the five gross elements.' Sound corresponds to ether or sky, the subtlest of the five material elements, which develop progressively from subtle to gross (ether, air, fire, water, earth). Sound is therefore the basis of all creation.

Hindu esoterics believe letters and words have four levels of meaning: physical, internal, vibrational (transmitted telepathically through *prana*) and transcendental. The Hebrew letter was considered to have at least three levels of influence: the inner structure of reality, physical nature and, finally, individual understanding and social communication.

Paul Von Ward, in his book *Gods, Genes, and Consciousness*, states that other cultures had similar views about the power of language. "Priests and shamans used primal sounds, producing an appropriate word to cause manifestation or action in the physical realm." He explains that "incantations and chants are examples of this belief, as are mantras[144] in Hinduism and Buddhism."

Von Ward surmises that if language has such power, then perhaps "we can learn to use words whose frequencies resonate with the energies of the desired effect."

Just as music is played externally and yet realized within, in the same way, words and their sounds have the power to vibrate to different parts of the body, different chakras, organs, and emotional and mental states. To a great degree, however, the efficacy of the sound is determined by the purity of the individual. Although the word or mantra already has a certain power, the way we enunciate the sound, our feelings, and the purpose behind the expression all have a major impact on its ultimate effect.

Every word we speak makes a thoughtform in the etheric and astral dimensions. Stewart Pearce[145] believes our voice can transform and enrich our life, because "the power of our voice crystalizes thought, and so its energy may be used to transmute our outlook, attitudes, beliefs, creativity, and physical presence ..." Our words literally draw the energy out of the subtle dimensions, crystallizing it into some manner of expression in the physical plane. If one is constantly exposed to negative words, their electromagnetic field (aura) can become permeated with such negative thoughtforms, causing others to feel uncomfortable in their presence.

An important part of the training within the ancient mystery schools was to control speech, including regulating words and their meanings. The importance of accuracy in reciting mantras within the Vedic tradition is one such example. If mantras are chanted improperly, they yield an opposite result. This happened when Tvasta performed a sacrifice to kill the great King Indra, as described in the *Bhagavat Purana*.

---

[144] *Sanskrit*: Consisting of two words, *man* (mind); *tra* (to deliver).
[145] *The Alchemy of Voice* p.19

Tvasta chanted a mantra to increase Indra's enemies, but because he chanted the mantra wrong, the sacrifice produced a demon of whom Indra was the enemy.[146]

Similarly, exaggerations and contradictory statements can create energetic blocks to manifesting our desires in the physical. A good rule is to take the time to thoroughly think through what you wish to say before actually saying it. Carefully consider the time, place and circumstance, and more importantly, the tone, inflection and correct pronunciation. Remember: sound creates.

Pure Sound

What is pure sound as opposed to impure sound? The answer to that question will depend largely on a person's world view and philosophical outlook. If you're a fan of industrial music, the screams of Emilie Autumn may be inspiring; for the poet, the prose of Shakespeare or Leonard Cohen may send shivers up your spine, and if you're a sci-fi geek, what better sound is there then the witty words of Doctor Who?

However, for the spiritualist, there is no more pure sound than the holy name of God. The Bible states:

Hallowed be thy name," and "In the beginning was the Word, and the Word was with God, and the Word was God. (John 1:1).

In the *Gita*, Krishna declares:

Of sacrifices I am the chanting of the holy names. (10.25).

Similarly, the holy Quran states:

His are the most beautiful names. (59.24).

Praising or chanting the name of God or the Goddess is a special form of prayer. In many religions, the excellence of

---

[146] *Bhagavat Purana* Verse: 6.9 summary

chanting the name(s) of God lies in the mystic syllables, which invoke God's purity and sovereign power. The various mantras in Hinduism and Buddhism – such as *Om, Hare Krishna, Namu-myo-ho-renge-kyo* or *Om Mane Padme Hum* – and the Roman Catholic practice of chanting on the Rosary all focus the mind on the spiritual plane and call forth its mystical elevating influence. In Christianity, prayers are offered in the name of Jesus Christ, who promises to do whatever is asked in faith. Indeed, in the hands of a great Adept, the power of transcendental sound to initiate change could conceivably be unlimited, when we consider that creation itself was but the result of the Spoken Word!

When we intone names of God and cause the name to vibrate throughout our body and consciousness, we align our energy with that aspect of the divine creative intelligence represented by the name.

A source for divine names for those that resonate with the Judeo-Christian tradition is the ancient Hebrew *Qabala*. The ten names contained in the Tree of Life are the ten manifestations of the divine within the physical world. Three names, Amen, Hu, and Eheieh are considered particularly effective.

But to play the devil's advocate here, the extraordinary effects produced by such prayer may also be a result of a principle described as sympathetic vibration. For example, if one of the wires of a harp is made to vibrate vigorously, its movement will affect a sympathetic vibration in the strings of other harps placed around it, if they are tuned to the same pitch. In other words, there is nothing transcendental going on here, just strings harmonizing by association. In any case, there is no doubt that after group prayer or focused group intention, powerful and transformative events do take place.

In the Jewish tradition the explicit name of God is too holy to be uttered by the human tongue. In particular, the Tetragrammaton YHWH, which is translated "the Lord" in modern Bibles, is never to be spoken. To show respect, God is often referred to paraphrastically by such terms as the Lord, Heaven, the King, the Almighty, the Name, and G-d. Thus, to praise and bless the name of God, as in the psalm quoted here, means to extol God's greatness and mighty works without mentioning His sacred name. The intention is always one of invoking a pure sound, and thus, an auspicious outcome.

Of special mention are traditions of the many names of God that enumerate His many attributes. The Qur'an contains the ninety-nine most beautiful names of Allah, and from the Mahabharata[147] there is the Vishnu sahasranama,[148] "the thousand names of Vishnu." Each name eulogizes one of Vishnu's countless great attributes. To recite these names, it is said, is to give a magnificent description of the height, depth, and breadth of divinity.

In the Sikh Adi Granth[149] it is stated:

> Contemplate solely the Name of God; fruitless are all other rituals. [150]

> The true essence, eternal is the Lord's Name. [151]

Probably the most famous mantra of Buddhism is Om mani padme hum, the six-syllable mantra of the Bodhisattva of compassion, Avalokiteshvara.[152] This mantra is particularly associated with the four-armed Shadakshari form of Avalokiteshvara. The Dalai Lama is said to be an incarnation

---

[147] Mahabharata is one of the two major Sanskrit epics of ancient India, the other being the Rāmāyana.

[148] The Vishnu sahasranama as found in the Mahabharata is the most popular version of the 1,000 names of Vishnu.

[149] The Adi Granth, literally "the first book," is the early compilation of the Sikh Scriptures by Sri Guru Arjan Dev Ji, the fifth Sikh Guru, in 1604.

[150] Sikhism. Adi Granth, Suhi, M.1, p. 728.

[151] Sikhism. Adi Granth, Gauri Sukhmani 19, M.5, p. 289.

[152] Avalokiteshvara (Tibetan: Chenrezig, Chinese: Guanyin).

of *Avalokiteshvara*, and so his devotees especially revere the mantra.

Further, in the Contemplation Sutra of Amitayus[153], it is stated:

> *If there be anyone who commits evil deeds... let him utter the name "Buddha Amitayus" serenely and with voice uninterrupted; let him be continually thinking of Buddha until he has completed ten times the thought, repeating, "Namu Amida Butsu." On the strength of uttering Buddha's name he will, during every repetition, expiate the sins. (3.30)*

Throughout the Vaisnava literature, the Maha Mantra (*Hare Krishna, Hare Krishna, Krishna Krishna, Hare Hare, Hare Rama, Hare Rama, Rama Rama, Hare Hare*) is praised for its efficacy to instill devotion to God and purify the chanter of all worldly desires.

One of the principle functions of the tongue is to vibrate, and therefore the great spiritual traditions of the world have always encouraged us to "praise the Lord." However, there are many other ways to purify the vibratory function of the tongue aside from prayer and reciting Holy Scripture; for example, speaking only palatable truths; speaking words that are beneficial to others, and expressing heart-felt gratitude.

Sri Krishna makes this clear when He states in verse 17.15 of the *Bhagavad-Gita*:

> *Austerity of speech consists in speaking words that are truthful, pleasing, beneficial, and not agitating to others, and also in regularly reciting Vedic literature[154].*

---

[153] One of the three major Buddhist *sutras* found within the Pure Land branch of Mahayana Buddhism.

[154] The *Sanksrit* term used here is *Svādhyāya* which has several meanings, including study of the *Vedas* and other sacred books, self-recitation, repetition of the *Vedas* aloud, and as a term for the *Vedas* themselves.

The 12th century saint, theologian and philosopher Ramanuja of the *Sri Sampradaya*, comments: "Words which consist totally of truth yet do not offend those spoken to and which are imbued with sweet and pleasing words that are inspiring and beneficial are austerities of speech in *sattva guna* (the mode of goodness).

Gratitude

Gratitude is a fruit of great cultivation; you do not find it among gross people – Samuel Johnson[155]

We must learn to be thankful for the blessings that surround us. It's so easy to find fault, but what do we achieve when we do that? Nothing, but unhappiness and frustration, with more of the same faulty behavior being attracted to us. It's better, therefore, to focus on what is right and wonderful in your life right now, for according to the "Law of Attraction," that sort of positive mindset will attract more of the same. The universe doesn't see negative or positive, after all; one man's poison is another man's nectar. In other words, because all thoughts are energy, and as Einstein proposed, mass is simply energy compressed, the thoughts we focus on become the building blocks of our physical reality. The bestselling books like *The Secret* popularized this concept, helping millions of people live more successful and fulfilling lives.

Milton[156] once wrote, "Gratitude bestows reverence, allowing us to encounter everyday epiphanies, those transcendent moments of awe that change forever how we experience life and the world."

This quote from Milton brings to mind a wonderful experience I once had in San Francisco.

---

[155] Samuel Johnson (English Poet, Critic and Writer. 1709-1784).

[156] John Milton (English Poet, Historian and Scholar. Ranks second, only to Shakespeare, among English poets. 1608-1674).

Café Gratitude

A lovely example of gratitude and positivity are the Café Gratitude restaurants in San Francisco, California, founded by Terces and Matthew Engelhart. Not only does the staff ooze with enthusiasm and appreciation, but even browsing the menu forces one to think positively about yourself and everyone at the table. Every item on the menu begins with the prefix "I am," and then lists entrees and drinks with superlatives like "lovely," "divine," "brilliant," "forgiving," "abundant," "joyful," etc. One cannot help but smile and feel good just reading the menu. It is a fantastic example for the entire restaurant industry. I remember feeling so blessed after eating there the first time, and then for the waitress to ask me, "So what are you thankful for today?" just capped off a truly divine experience.

Consider the practical benefits of a positive and grateful attitude: it will make you and those around you happier, or at the very least, it will help you to not get distracted by frivolous and unproductive behavior. So what can we lose by adopting a positive and thankful attitude? Nothing at all – but the gains are immense and tangible. Unfortunately, complaining and blaming others for the difficulties in our lives has become an all too common characteristic of modern society. Why so? Because misery loves company. When we feel defeated, in a desperate attempt to create normality in our life, we search for meaning and relevance. The easiest way to do this is to "level the playing field" and do whatever is necessary to bring the world down to our level of awareness. Often this takes the form of justifying our mistakes or shirking the responsibility, and in doing so, we typically ignore the blessings that surround us, or possibly the lessons to be gained.

Worse still is to assume superiority by pushing others down. The entire capitalist model is fueled by the need to usurp, cheat, or inconvenience someone else. Of course, I am not suggesting that business can never be conducted with an attitude of gratitude; however, to consistently succeed necessitates marginalizing or immobilizing competition.

The news industry operates on a similar model. Bad news sells. We watch the news to learn about the misfortune of others, because, in a diabolical way, it gives us a sense of relief knowing that the misfortune did not befall us.

Try this experiment today. Go out of your way to tell a stranger or a colleague how important and appreciative you are of their service to their family, community or friends. For example, when you get out of the taxi or bus, look the person in the eye and say, "Thank you for serving me," and really mean it. Make them believe your sincerity. Do the same to the person at your local grocery store; to your UPS man and, heaven forbid, the police officer that pulls you over. I did this once after the officer let me off for speeding. I looked him in the eye and said, "Thank you for making the roads safer." I sincerely meant what I said, and I could see that it took him by surprise and he really appreciated it. It made me feel great too.

It is so easy to find fault in this world. After all, it is not designed to be a place of permanence but rather more like a developmental phase for the spirit, or a kind of "hospital for the soul." Consequently, the humans that fill the "wards" of this mundane world are sickly and imperfect. So rather than point out the obvious, take the divine path and look for the beauty in all. Be like the honeybee and seek the "nectar" or the good in everything and everyone, and avoid at all cost acting like a fly that seeks out the rotten imperfections in everything. A "fly" mentality will only attract negativity.

LIVING IN THE MOMENT

It is said that you can't change the past, but you can ruin the present by worrying about the future. One day, while lying in bed, I spent many hours just recalling past childhood memories, looking for answers to the question "What made me the person I am today?" The exercise was certainly interesting, and yet despite how hard I tried, all I got were the same old memories. I visualized myself walking around my old house and then in the homes of friends and relatives, all the while trying to stimulate the mind for new pictures and experiences that I could learn from. However, no matter how hard I tried, I found nothing really compelling or instructive, other than what I already had come to realize about myself thus far.

But then it struck me that all those past memories are just that: memories – or mental photographs and video – that no longer exist. They are illusory and gone forever. Yes, they serve a function of supporting the philosophical paradigm I currently adopt, but other than that, they're useless. What really matters is what is happening *now*? Who am I *now*? What can I be thankful for *now*? What do I want *now*?

As I meditated on the *now*, it reinforced the importance of steering clear of meditating on what I don't want. Too often we think and speak about what we don't want to happen, or what we don't like, rather than what we actually want to happen or appreciate. Such thoughts and discussions are not only unproductive, but can actually be incredibly harmful. You see, by thinking and talking about what you don't want, you're in effect attracting that very thing to you. As explained in the previous chapters, the vibrations you send out in the form of words and mental thoughts act like a magnet, compelling the Universe to send those projected experiences your way.

The Intention Experiment

Lynne McTaggart, international bestselling author of *The Intention Experiment*, was asked about the power of negative thought and what to do about it:

> *I like the work of Dr. John Diamond, who was the father of behavioral kinesiology. He found that there's only one thing that prevents people from being weakened by negative thoughts, and that is what he calls the "homing thought," which is the sense of what you were put on this earth to do. It's the thing you do that transcends everything. If you keep that in mind when you're bombarded by someone's negative thoughts that makes you strong.*

In *The Intention Experiment*, McTaggart narrates the exciting developments in the science of intention. She also profiles the colorful scientists and renowned pioneers who study the effects of focused group intention on scientifically quantifiable targets – animal, plant, and human.

Citing cutting-edge research conducted at Princeton, MIT, Stanford, and many other prestigious universities and laboratories, *The Intention Experiment* reveals that a vast quantum energy field connects the universe. Thought generates its own palpable energy, which you can use to improve your life and, when you are harnessed with an interconnected group, to change the world.

Reading *The Intention Experiment* forced me to rethink what it means to be human. It proved to me in very scientific terms just how connected I am to everyone and everything around me, and this discovery demanded that I pay better attention to my thoughts, intentions, and actions.

Soon after, I began my days meditating on what I wanted in my life and what I could be thankful for right *now*. It is an exercise we should do every morning because it sets a positive framework for the rest of the day.

Living in the *now* is really all that matters. Our lives are, in essence, just a collection of *now* moments, strung together in an illusory garland of time. In the higher spiritual planes, there *is* no time. Time is conspicuous by its absence. Life in the spiritual realm is eternal, so the concepts of past, present and future do not exist. Spiritual existence is all about *now*.

Learning to live in the moment is truly a gift of immeasurable worth. In the Western world, we are brainwashed to think in terms of schedules and deadlines, so our lives sometimes feel like a blur of unfulfilled experiences. The word "deadline" seems to solidify the idea that we are racing against the clock to meet our death!

Take a moment to stop and study the faces of people during rush hour and notice how anxious and worried they appear. The consumer-driven system we have adopted in the West keeps us running on a treadmill going nowhere. And there is another interesting word: "nowhere." It can also be written as *now here*. Instead of running for some mirage in the future, it is better to stop and appreciate what is *now here*. **The most basic form of gratitude** is appreciating the blessing of food in your life.

The last 12 months of my life have probably been as transforming to me as the year I became a monk way back in 1983. At that time, as now, I began deconstructing everything I had ever learned up to that point and building a new reality for myself. Shaving my head back then was a big part of that experience. I remember looking in the mirror and thinking how different I looked, and that all of the vanity that came with those long locks was now lying on the floor ready to be swept away. I felt so liberated. A new persona had emerged. I was "born again," if you will. From that day on, I dove deeply into the devotional path of *bhakti* yoga and never once regretted that decision.

So much has happened since that fateful day 28 years ago. Such is life, that despite our best efforts to create permanence, we are constantly subjected to change, willingly or unwillingly. The only way to navigate these challenges is to always remain objective and embrace the lessons learned. The new *me* living in the *now*, although still strongly drawing on my experience as a *Vaisnava* monk, is a work in progress as I appreciate other spiritual traditions and honor and respect the perspective and opinions of great thinkers, philosophers, adherents, and even antagonists of these traditions.

Unique and Divine

The important thing to realize is that ultimately we are not Christian, Hindu, Vaisnava, Muslim, Zoroastrian, Jewish, or Buddhist, all of which are just superficial designations; rather, we simply are. You and I are unique individuals. There is no need to put a label on *who* you are. Nor is there a need to define you by some church, temple, synagogue, community, gender, race or religion. You are who you are -a fragment of the splendor of God. We are actually little gods and goddesses having a human experience. Commentator of the *Gita*, Srila Prabhupada explains:

> *The entire cosmic manifestations, moving and nonmoving, are manifested by different activities of Krishna's energy. In the material existence we create different relationships with different living entities who are nothing but Krishna's marginal energy, but under the creation of prakrti[157] some of them appear as our father, mother, grandfather, creator, etc., but actually they are parts and parcels of Krishna. As such, these living entities who appear to be our father, mother, etc., are nothing but Krishna. In this verse the word dhata means "creator." Not only are our father and mother parts and parcels of Krishna, but their creator, grandmother, and grandfather, etc., are also Krishna. Actually any living entity, being part and parcel of Krishna, is Krishna[158].*

---

[157] *Sanskrit, prakrti*: Material Nature.
[158] *Bhagavad-gita As It Is* (Purport Verse 9.17).

Each one of us will go through life experiencing the world in our unique way. No two people will have the same experience and no two people will ever have the same conclusion. Even if only slight, the "flavor" of that experience will always be different from one person to the next. And there lies one of the fundamental wonders of this universe. Yes, we are all connected; yes, we all emanate from the same energetic source; yes, we are all ultimately heading in the same direction, but amazingly we are all still absolutely unique individuals.

It is this tapestry of individualism that makes the life experience so astonishing. In the same way that each brush stroke of a painting; each tile within a mosaic; each flower within a garden; each star in the firmament; each thread in a gorgeous gown; or each note in a symphony all work together to create something magical – each one of us is a participant in the play of life and together, connected by the loving energy that brought us forth. We have the inherent ability to transform, uplift and create something even more wonderful for our own life and the life of others.

Your human experience is meant to facilitate self-discovery, bringing you to the point where you will absolutely know who you are on the highest spiritual planes of existence. That search begins with recognizing that you are an eternal spiritual being, far more significant than some gross physical body. Once you are established in this divine paradigm, characterized by the absence of time, you then need to focus all your thoughts, gratitude and actions on what is happening now, because in absolute reality, now is all that really matters.

When death comes knocking on your door, the only thing you can hold onto is the present moment and how you are responding to it. To live in the moment is to live eternally.

THE GIFT OF FOOD

Tell me what you eat, and I will tell you what you are.
- Anthelme Brillat-Savarin[159]

Food as a Medium of LOVE

Whether the holiday is *Thanksgiving, Christmas, Easter, Hanukah, Janmastami,* or *Diwali,* you can be sure that there is plenty of feasting and lots of joy in the air. Indeed, none of these public holidays or religious festivals would be complete without the sharing of sumptuous food in a loving atmosphere. Food is one of the universally accepted ways that we express love for one another. Unfortunately, these festive holidays are often celebrated at the expense of innocent animals' lives. It does not have to be that way, but due to ignorance, misinformation or just plain lust, people choose to eat slaughtered animals or products made as a result of animal cruelty on these joyous occasions.

I remember the first time I attended a Christmas party with friends in Sydney, Australia, after turning vegetarian and how shocked I was to see a pig's leg on the table. I asked my friend, "Do you know there is a corpse on your table?" He looked at me incredulously and said, "Oh come on, it's just a leg of ham!" Exactly. What gives us the right to eat another living being's leg when there are so many other options?

Look at any supermarket aisle; there are literally thousands of non-violent foods to choose from and yet the common misconception (fueled by the meat and dairy industry) is that a vegetarian subsists on carrots and lettuce alone.

---

[159] Jean Anthelme Brillat-Savarin (1755–1826, Paris) was a French lawyer and politician who gained fame as an epicure and gastronome.

Even if you are attached to the taste of meat and dairy, food technology has advanced so much over the last two decades that mock meats and mock dairy products fill entire sections of the supermarket, from "fish fillets," to "steaks," "hot dogs," and melting "cheeses" all made with non-animal ingredients, but so authentic that they can fool even a hard-core carnivore. However, be warned, because a recent investigation in Los Angeles revealed that some of these "mock meats" coming out of Taiwan actually contained animal extracts.[160] If you want to eat an entirely plant-based diet, therefore, with no chance of contamination by animal-derived ingredients, the only solution is to grow your own food and prepare it at home, seed to plate.

You Have a Choice

The food choices you make say much about the kind of love and respect you have for the world. Despite your good intentions, if the expression of your love comes at the expense of an innocent animal's life, your offering is impure. Food, like water, carries a vibration, and a slaughtered animal's corpse is filled with fear, anger, pain, and sadness. That same energy is absorbed into every cell of your body when you consume such rotting flesh. How, then, can we truly celebrate these festive holidays, glorified as days of light, love and hope, by passing around scorched or baked rotting flesh? To do so is hypocritical and unjustifiable.

Unfortunately, we've become lazy slaves to convenience. It is just too easy to follow these bogus traditions and not rock the boat. Is it not far nobler to act on the principle of love and light and set an example for our children and friends? It takes a brave person to raise his head above the crowd and take a stand for the innocent.

---

[160] *Operation Pancake*: an undercover investigation of LA vegan restaurants was conducted by Quarry Girl and reported on her blog in June 2009.

Food Unites

In this world, there is no greater medium than food to unite people of conflicting natures. Whether the difference is philosophical, political or even dietary, just about everyone will put aside differences to come together and eat. Such is the power of food.

It is on this understanding that the Vedic culture of hospitality is based. Food in its most pure form is the best conduit to express respect and love to every living being. Indeed, it seems that food speaks a universal language of love that everyone can understand, even the deaf, dumb and blind.

It must be pointed out that it is not actually the physical substance of food that has the power to unite, but rather the intention that it carries. Even food that is considered ignorant, like the rotting flesh of an animal or food that has been contaminated by a plethora of artificial ingredients, can still have some power to create unity if only temporarily – *if* it is infused with loving intention. This is clearly evident during holidays like Christmas. However, the unifying effects are short lived as any good intention is quickly overwhelmed by the feelings of fear, pain and sadness of the animal that are also present in the meat.

For the most lasting and transformative effect, food needs to be completely free of any negative karma. The purest food is that food that has been not only prepared with loving intention, but also offered with love to the source from which it came – God.

Author and filmmaker, David Wilcock believes that by investing positive energy into food we can make it more healthful for ourselves and others, "*You can change the structure of your own food by intent...That's why it is so important to bless your food, because you can take the existing stuff you are already using and make it much more potent, by making it yours, by putting your energy into it.*"

How does Food Carry Intention?

Because food is mostly water (the most powerful conduit of thought energy), all food is in one way or another impacted by how it is grown, handled, packaged, prepared, cooked and served. Every person who interacts with a food on its journey from seedling to your plate intrinsically affects the food's energetic quality, and subsequently your physical, mental and spiritual health. Each person's thoughts (psychic energy) add to the palette of conscious thoughts that eventually makes their way into your body.

It is no surprise, then, that we sometimes have terrible dreams or feel uneasy, depressed or mentally clouded after eating out. Do you really know what goes on behind those closed kitchen doors? Do you even know who is preparing your meals, or what standard of life they lead? Probably not. So, if you truly wish to raise your consciousness to the highest level, avoid eating out altogether, or at the very least, be very selective and make an effort to know the people who are preparing your meals and what standards of hygiene they employ and what their standard of food selection is. Otherwise, when you eat out you're literally 'throwing the dice' on your mental, physical and spiritual health.

The *Chaitanya Charitamrita* puts it this way:

> *When one eats food prepared by an impure person, one's mind becomes impure, and when the mind is thus contaminated, one is unable to think of Krishna (God).*[161]

A food yogi will always make the extra effort to protect their mental well-being. "Mental health is an integral part of health; indeed, there is no health without mental health," declares the World Health Organization (WHO).

---

[161] CC *Antya Lila* Verse 6.278 (edited for clarity).

Thought Toxins

Most people will not concern themselves with the potential dangers of "thought toxins" in their meals, but considering how mentally sick people are these days, we should be. For example, according to a report[162] released by The Mental Health Foundation in UK, "Changes in diet over the past 50 years appear to be an important factor behind a significant rise in mental ill health in the UK." The Mental Health Foundation claims, "Scientific studies have clearly linked attention deficit disorder, depression, Alzheimer's disease and schizophrenia to junk food and the absence of essential fats, vitamins and minerals in industrialized diets."

A further report,[163] published by the non-profit Sustain,[164] states that the modern fast food diet is "fuelling not only obesity, cardiovascular disease, diabetes and some cancers, but may also be contributing to rising rates of mental ill-health and anti-social behavior."

According to WHO, more than 450 million people suffer from mental disorders worldwide.[165]

Physical Toxins

In the US alone, the Centers for Disease Control (CDC) estimates that over 1,800 people die each year from pathogens transmitted via food. To be fair, however, not all these cases are a result of eating out, as illustrated by the crisis at Maple Leaf Foods (Canada), in which packaged meat products

---

[162] Report: *Diet and Mental Health*: January 16th, 2006.

[163] *How are food and mental health related?*: April 9, 2010.

[164] SUSTAIN is a non-profit alliance of 100 national public interest organizations lobbying for better food and agricultural policies and practices to enhance the health and welfare of people and animals, improve the working and living environment, enrich society and culture and promote equity.

[165]*Mental health: strengthening our response* (report 202): September, 2010

contaminated by listeria bacteria were shipped to grocery stores.

In any case, food poisoning is the result of eating food contaminated with bacteria such as staphylococcus or E. coli, typically found in low vibration foods like rotting flesh and contaminated dairy products – yet another reason to stick with the more *sattvic*, higher vibration and organic, plant-based diet. However, E. coli can sometimes contaminate safe foods, like spinach, when farmers use contaminated manure-based fertilizers on crops. The negligence of these farmers carries over into the vegetable crop to create an inferior plant species that is not only potentially harmful to physical health, but also damaging to our mental well-being.

Thanksgiving – a Day to Honor All Life

In the US, Thanksgiving is a time when families and friends come together to reaffirm their love and appreciation for one another through the age-old custom of sharing food. As mentioned earlier, Americans will eat more than 50 million turkeys on this day.

Why do Americans think it necessary to slaughter so many innocent animals to show their love for each other? It is a sad commentary on modern society that we have so much to be thankful for, and yet we carve up innocent animals on major holidays to express that sentiment. And at what expense? Americans are getting fatter and sicker year after year. The three top causes of death – heart disease, cancer and diabetes – are all food related. Eating a greasy, fat-laden dead bird is not going to help matters. But millions do it anyway, in the name of tradition.

The origins of the Thanksgiving celebration are not as blessed as most people think. Thanksgiving is a quintessentially American holiday, so much so that it is often considered one of their holy days and is almost universally celebrated by Americans around the world. Ironically, in truth, American families get together to celebrate one genocide (against Native Americans) by committing another genocide (against turkeys). How can people celebrate in good faith and conscience?

On Thanksgiving Day, Americans give thanks for being the invader, the exploiter, the greedy, the colonizer, the thief, indeed the *genocidaire*. As Mark Twain points out in his *War Prayer*:

> *Wishing and being thankful for one's own success and victory is, at the very same time, wishing and being thankful for another's defeat and destruction.*

Do Americans really want to make these kinds of wishes and give these kinds of thanks?

I do not wish to belabor the disturbing history that Thanksgiving represents, mainly because most people reading this book will probably already be vegetarian and much more conscious in their eating habits. On Thanksgiving, however, I urge one and all to be consistent with the true spirit of the holiday by sharing pure food with love and respect for all of God's creation. Do not conform to the bogus traditions perpetrated by self-serving corporations, but rather stand strong on principle, and make this day a day where you honor God and all creation for what it truly is - your larger spiritual family.

Food in its purest form has the power to unite and heal and, more importantly, to create real peace and prosperity in the world. I believe that such food, given in a spirit of love, is the solution to all problems simply because food is so central to every cultural gathering, every spiritual holiday, every ritual, every battle, and every celebration - and, of course, because without food there is no meaning to life.

Thanksgiving, therefore, should be a day that highlights the importance of food in our lives and how critical it is to our physical, mental, spiritual and cultural health. By eating flesh, we defile this holiday and lose touch with the very spirit of giving thanks. By taking the life of another, we offend God's creation and abuse the blessings human life affords us.

Instead of eating a turkey, we should invite a turkey to dinner and feed it as we would any other animate being that came asking for a meal.

The Farm Animal Reform Movement (FARM) has this to say:

> *Abusing and killing an innocent bird betrays the life-affirming spirit of giving thanks for our life, health, and happiness. The nearly 300 million turkeys killed each year in the US spend their entire lives crammed in large sheds with little room to move. Artificially inseminated and selectively bred to gain enormous amounts of weight, they suffer heart attacks, broken limbs, lameness, and death from their genetically-induced accelerated growth rate. Most of these same conditions apply to "free range" turkeys.*

Let the madness and hypocrisy stop once and for all.

Popular conscious musician *Human* wrote the following song that beautifully captures the sad history of the American genocide of native Indians, while at the same time making a heart-warming plea for all of us to realize just how connected we all are, despite the apparent differences on the surface. The song features on the *Breathe* album by *The Human Revolution* band.

Don't Ignore

Broken treaties, stolen lives, mislead the children
and the culture won't survive.
Cannot be trusted, poisoned with greed,
disgrace the mother, watch her people bleed.

Seems like things never change,
Same rich white men playin' the same old game,
It ain't a color its a way of life,
Keepin the poor and the colored underneath the knife.

It's the way of money, it's the way of greed,
Exploit the earth, pollute the water,

sell what they don't need,
The 4-leggeds livin' on the land,
Become another possession in the white man's hands.

It don't matter who we're related to,
We all come from the same religious group,
We have similar wants, we have the same needs,
We all wanna survive, we all have to eat.

Its time we all help each other out,
Cooperation's in, competitions out,
We better start to turn things around,
Put your ear to the ground, you hear that tremblin' sound.

It's the Earth Mother gonna start pushin' back,
All these smokes stacks givin' her a heart attack,
You can't take her blood without givin' back,
You leave holes in the ground while above her skin cracks.

But she's so strong, she'll live on,
Long after we're all dead and gone.
Its not too late to turn it all around,
Change is the name of the game in this song.

Ain't no shame in bein' proud of where you come from,
But don't ignore the history,
Millions will never know who their ancestor were,
But we can begin to set these tortured people free.

It's time we rewrite these Babylon books,
It's time to give history a second look,
And stop ignoring what our ancestors have done,
So many have died by their blankets and guns.

We can't give back all the stolen lives,
But we can heal the past, we can finally cry,
And vow that it won't ever happen again,
We can learn from the past, start making amends.

And give sovereignty back to their tribes,
Prove we have honor, repent for our lies,

Stop diggin' up the burial grounds,
Restore their languages and rename the towns.

Cause they were here first, we owe it to them,
We must protect them from our own government,
I can't understand why they don't leave 'em alone,
All the meat is gone, all that's left is bone.

And I declare right now, till the day I die,
That I won't watch this injustice happen through my eyes,
It's the same with Iraq, its the same all around,
This sick culture must finally fall to the ground.

Broken treaties, stolen lives, mislead the children and the culture won't survive.

Cannot be trusted, poisoned with greed, disgrace the mother, watch her people bleed.

Don't Ignore. © Copyright 2006 Human

Compassion for Animals

Reverend Andrew Linzey suggests in his book, *Love the Animals*, that a compassionate sensitivity towards animals is inseparable from the proclamation of the Christian Gospel: "We have lived so long with the Gospel stories of Jesus that we frequently fail to see how his life and ministry identified with animals almost at every point. His birth, if tradition is to be believed, takes place in the home of sheep and oxen. His ministry begins, according to St. Mark, in the wilderness 'with the wild beasts' (1:13). His triumphal entry into Jerusalem involved riding on a 'humble' ass (Matthew 21). According to Jesus, it is lawful to 'do good' on the Sabbath, which includes the rescuing of an animal fallen into a pit (Matthew 12). Even the sparrows, literally sold for a few pennies in his day, are not 'forgotten before God.' God's providence extends to the entire created order and the glory of Solomon and all his works cannot be compared to that of the lilies of the field (Luke 12:27)."

"It is a loving heart which is required by God, and not needless bloodletting of God's creatures," concludes Linzey. "It is 'the merciful' who are 'blessed' in God's sight and what we do to 'the least' of all we do to him (Matthew 5:7, 25:45-46).

According to the Mahayana Buddhist tradition, "The eating of meat extinguishes the seed of great compassion.[166]"

Many Georgian saints were distinguished by their love for animals. For example, St. John Zedazneli made friends with bears near his hermitage; St. Shio befriended a wolf; St. David of Garesja protected birds and deer from hunters, proclaiming, 'He whom I believe in and worship looks after and feeds all these creatures.' Similarly, some early Celtic saints favored compassion for animals. Saint Wales, Cornwall

---

[166] *Mahaparinirvana sutra.*

and Brittany of Ireland in the 5th and 6th centuries AD healed and prayed for animals.

St. Francis of Assisi (1182–1226) felt a deep kinship with all animals, calling them "brother" and "sister," knowing they came form the same Source as himself.

Christian mystic, Thomas A' Kempis (1380–1471) wrote in his devotional classic, *The Imitation of Christ*, that the soul desiring communion with God must be open to seeing, respecting and learning from all of God's creatures, including the nonhumans:

> *...and if thy heart be straight with God, then every creature shall be to thee a mirror of life and a book of holy doctrine, for there is no creature so little or vile, but that showeth and representeth the goodness of God.*

Roman Catholic priest, Reverend Basil Wrighton stated in 1965:

> *To stand for Christ is to stand against the evil of cruelty inflicted on those who are weak, vulnerable, unprotected, undefended, morally innocent, and in that class we must unambiguously include animals....Look around you and see the faces of Christ in the millions of innocent animals suffering in factory farms, in laboratories, in abattoirs, in circuses and in animals hunted for sport.*

The *Atharva Veda*[167] emphatically states that only those who respect animals can be considered serious spiritual practitioners:

> *Those noble souls who practice meditation and other yogic ways, who are ever careful about all beings, who protect all animals, are the ones who are actually serious about spiritual practices.*

---

[167] Verse 19.48.5.

The Karma connection

Srila Prabhupada, the founder of Food for Life, believed that human wars are the direct result of slaughtering innocent animals. For example, in 1973, he wrote in a *Bhagavat Purana* commentary to verse 4.26.5:

In this age of Kali the propensity for mercy is almost nil. Consequently there is always fighting and wars between men and nations. Men do not understand that because they unrestrictedly kill so many animals, they also must be slaughtered like animals in big wars. This is very much evident in the Western countries. In the West, slaughterhouses are maintained without restriction, and therefore every fifth or tenth year there is a big war in which countless people are slaughtered even more cruelly than the animals.

Furthermore, in his commentary to verse 6.10.9 he stated:

One cannot continue killing and at the same time be a religious man. That is the greatest hypocrisy. Jesus Christ said, 'Do not kill,' but hypocrites nevertheless maintain thousands of slaughterhouses while posing as Christians.

Russian philosopher Leo Tolstoy[168] concurred:

By killing, man suppresses in himself, unnecessarily, the highest spiritual capacity, that of sympathy and pity towards living creatures like himself and by violating his own feelings becomes cruel. As long as there are slaughterhouses, there will be battlefields.

On days like Thanksgiving and Christmas this wholesale human karma is elevated to astronomical proportions, thus paving the way for more suffering. There may not be much one person can do to change the collective karma of the

---

[168] Leo Nikolayevich Tolstoy (1828-1910) was a Russian writer of realist fiction and philosophical essays.

masses that defile these holiday celebrations, but if you choose to reject these bogus killing traditions, you can at least feel satisfied that you did not contribute to the chaos that is created day after day. You will be one step closer to living with full integrity and realizing your spiritual connection to the world around you.

GOING BEYOND DIET

Until he extends the circle of his compassion to all living things, man will not himself find peace.
– Albert Schweitzer[169]

Oprah Winfrey has been embroiled in her fair share of controversy when it comes to dieting. The famous TEXAS CATTLEMEN vs. HOWARD LYMAN & OPRAH WINFREY case (1996) is one such example. More recently, inspired by Kathy Freston's book *Quantum Wellness*, Oprah embarked on a 21-day cleanse and hired vegan chef Tal Ronnen to prepare meals for her. In the early stages of her vegan fast, Oprah said: "Well, I feel like I got baptized in Vegan Land today....Wow, wow, wow! I never imagined meatless meals could be so satisfying."

At the completion of her fast, Oprah had a new appreciation for a plant-based lifestyle and, more importantly, she had discovered how to be more appreciative of food in general:

> *What I know for sure is I've reached a new level of awareness about food, eating and the whole process of how it gets to my table. I used to say thanks before a meal out of perfunctory habit. Now I consider it true grace to be able to eat anything in a world of increasing food shortages and starving people.*

Remembering her humble roots, Oprah told the story of how her grandmother grew and harvested everything: "Going to the garden was something I took for granted...now it thrills me to see the baskets of lettuce, fava beans, and herbs, fresh picked."

---

[169] Albert Schweitzer, German-French philosopher, physician, and musician (Nobel 1952).

In conclusion, she stated: "This has been exactly what we intended: enlightening. I will forever be a more cautious and conscious eater. That's my commitment for now. To stay awakened."

A Plant-Based Diet Is Not Enough

I did not become a vegetarian for my health; I did it for the health of the chickens. — Isaac Bashevis Singer

Subsisting on a plant-based diet is not the epitome of puritanical gorging. Pigeons, monkeys, elephants, koalas and a host of other wildlife subsist on a plant-based diet, so as members of the so-called "higher race," we should do more. It is astonishing how many vegans and vegetarians are convinced that diet alone will guarantee their successful spiritual evolution.

Evolution of the spirit is not exclusively tied to dietary preferences, although diet certainly does play a fundamental role. According to the *Vedas*, before incarnating into a human form, the soul transmigrates through millions of bodies – "8.4 million," states the *Bhagavat Purana*. Indeed, it appears that the soul rides on a perpetual reincarnation "ferris wheel" until it finally qualifies for a human birth. More importantly, only through the human experience is the soul capable of escaping this seemingly unending cycle. Although it is possible for animals to express divine realization and transcend this mundane world, it is indeed rare. Nonetheless, the human form and the human condition are especially equipped for the acquisition of higher spiritual knowledge. If we so desire and are karmically qualified, such higher spiritual knowledge can free us from the shackles of reincarnation.

Granted, a plant-based diet is the *foundation* for a higher human experience, but eating for health alone, without any consideration for the morality of a plant-based diet, will not awaken our full spiritual potential. Consuming food that is lower on the food chain and of a higher vibration, as well as less karmically entangling, will no doubt, over time, gradually purify one's consciousness and provide the bedrock for higher dimensional realizations. It just may not be sufficient for one lifetime, and that is something any student of metaphysics should be concerned with.

Karma-free Vegan

Because there is some form of violence even in the gathering and preparation of vegan meals, no food is ever totally karma-free, or *ahimsa* (non-violent) unless it is first offered in gratitude to God, at which time it becomes pure, antiseptic, and spiritually nourishing. By adopting this spiritual practice, a vegan can further their quest for real peace, harmony and spiritual purity. Despite our good intentions, if we fail to recognize God/Goddess as the source of all creation, our efforts will remain dry, mundane and inadequate.

Mother's Love

God could not be everywhere, so he created mothers.
- Jewish Proverb

Nothing can compare to a home-cooked meal from a loving mother. We've already talked about the risk we take with our emotional, physical and spiritual well-being when we eat out. Well, in the ideal home, a mother's cooking is filled with loving intention and healing energy and is therefore *the best* source of spiritual and physical nutrition on the planet! (Of course, with modern gender roles so blurred, the same could be said of a loving father!)

The sad truth, however, is that with mothers all over the world ceding control of the dinner table to scientists, food marketers and governments, a terrible thing happened. Tradition and commonsense went out the window, and as Michael Pollan notes, "Thirty years of nutritional advice have left us fatter, sicker, and more poorly nourished. Which is why we find ourselves in the predicament we do: in need of a whole new way to think about eating.[170]"

A loving nurturer like a mother will invest all her loving intention into the meals she prepares. That sort of loving intention is not only invaluable, but also worshipable. In fact, in the Vedic tradition, the father (*Pitru Devo Bhavaa*) and mother (*Matru Devo Bhavaa*) are considered the first guru and second guru respectively and should therefore be worshipped.

In Sanskrit, the word "guru" consists of two words: "*gu*" – which means darkness or ignorance and "*ru*" which means "remover of." The guru is someone who helps to remove ignorance from our hearts and enlightens us.

In the Bible, it is also stated:

> *Honor thy father and mother; which is the first commandment with promise; that it may be well with thee, and thou mayest live long on the earth.*

I have provided a comparison chart between food prepared by a loving Mother and that which you can buy in a restaurant. I could have extended this list indefinitely, but these are what I feel to be the most important pros and cons of eating a meal prepared by one's loving mother versus a meal prepared by a restaurant:

---

[170] *In Defense of Food*, Michael Pollen p 81.

Prepared by a loving mother	Prepared at a restaurant
Made with loving intention	Made with the intention of profit
Prepared carefully	Prepared hastily
Cleanliness honored	Cleanliness compromised
Selfless	Selfish
Focused intention	Distracted intention
Pure motivation	Material motivation

It is easy to see the benefits of eating a home cooked meal, and yet, every year, Americans will spend, on average, $1,000 eating out (which is said to be less than it once was).

Good Magazine, in partnership with Whole Foods, chronicled[171] the proportion of income Americans spend on food today as compared to the past. And guess what? They're spending less than ever.

In 1949, Americans spent 22% of their incomes on food, whereas in 2009 they spent a meager 10%. However, of this 10%, nearly half (40%)[172] is spent on food away from home, and research[173] has found that meals prepared outside the home are less healthful.

How is this so? Because, while saving money seems like a good thing, the cheap processed foods we buy outside are often produced by factory farming and industrial agriculture and supported by government subsidies, which we ultimately pay for in the form of taxes. Also, with jumbo-sized products being priced more economically, Americans may be getting

---

[171] Source: http://www.youtube.com/watch?v=reyxkSWUjLI&.

[172] US. Department of Labor, US Bureau of Labor Statistics, Consumer Expenditures in 2007 (Washington DC 2009).

[173] J.F.Guthrie, B.H. Lin, and E Frazao, Role of food prepared away from home in the American diet, 1977-78 versus 1994-96: Changes and consequences, J Nutr Educ Behav 34 (2002): 140-50.

more for their dollar, but they're also gaining more weight, losing their health, spending more on healthcare, and supporting environmentally unsustainable practices.

The Seven Mothers

According to the Vedic tradition, there are actually seven mothers in our life:

The first mother is our biological mother, from whose womb we have come to this world. Then there is the wife of the teacher or spiritual master; the wife of a priest; the wife of the king, or the queen; the cow; the nurse or caregiver; and, finally, the earth, often referred to as "Mother Nature." In Sanskrit, the country in which we take birth is called *desa matrika* or "motherland." We refer to our language as "mother tongue." So you can see that there are so many mothers, including the cow, in the Hindu tradition, because of her selfless service to provide milk. In India, a cow is sometimes addressed as *amba*, which also means mother.

There is one common principle that characterizes all genuine mothers, and that is selfless, loving service to their dependents. This pure loving intention is the true life-giving force that our mothers nurture us with. Whether it is milk from her breast or the fruit of a tree, a mother's offering is pure. No matter how hard modern science tries to emulate the pure offering of a mother, it will never succeed. The failed history of baby formula is a case in point. In a recent report by the Environmental Working Group (EWG), tests performed on liquid baby formulas found that they all contained *bisphenol A* (BPA). All major baby formula manufacturers use this leaching, hormone-mimicking chemical in the linings of the metal cans in which baby formula is sold.

BPA has been found to cause hyperactivity, reproductive abnormalities and pediatric brain cancer in lab animals. Increasingly, scientists suspect that BPA might be linked to several medical problems in humans, including breast and testicular cancer.

Food is a gift from MOTHER Earth

Humans cannot actually manufacture food. We can manipulate ingredients, but it is impossible for us to create food from scratch. Of course you could plant a seed and cultivate a garden, but who created the seed? Within every seed lies a dormant plant or tree, ready to fruit and spread more seed. The phenomenon is an endless cycle of kinetic transmutation of nature, to which Man has little to do with. American Playwright, George Bernard Shaw put it this way:

> *Think of the fierce energy concentrated in an acorn! You bury it in the ground, and it explodes into an oak! Bury a sheep, and nothing happens but decay.*

Despite technological advances in food production, including cloning and genetic manipulation of foods, genetic scientists have failed to create a single blade of grass from raw chemicals. Genetic engineering (GE) and genetically modified organisms (GMO) are, in reality, just modifications of what has already been naturally created by Mother Nature. It is absurd to think that we can ever match the brilliance of Mother Nature and create like her.

Offering Food Back to the Creators

The beginning of true human evolution comes when we acknowledge this dependence on the Great Creators (the Divine Masculine and the Divine Feminine) and begin to offer our food to them with gratitude and love. Only when we understand our innate connection to our Creators can we begin to experience genuine happiness and contentment, just as a fish does when returned to water, its natural environment. By offering food back to our Source with loving intention, we acknowledge our dependence on a higher power, while expressing our gratitude in a practical way. For example, when a young child offers her parents a "work of art" with sincere love, the parents naturally accept the offering of love with gratitude. No God or Goddess requires our humble offering, but they *will* accept the loving energy invested in it with great satisfaction. This symbiotic and dynamic reciprocation of love is what energizes and maintains the entire creation.

American marine biologist and nature writer, Rachel Louise Carson,[174] whose writings are credited with advancing the global environmental movement, once said:

> *Those who contemplate the beauty of the earth find reserves of strength that will endure as long as life lasts.*

"The beauty of the earth" is more than her external display of creative brilliance. Mother Earth serves us day after day, selflessly producing everything we need to survive. By appreciating her loving actions day after day we align our consciousness with the most powerful energy in the Universe – love. One way to appreciate and reciprocate that selfless love is by adopting the "Food Yogi Diet."

---

[174] Rachel Louise Carson (May 27, 1907 – April 14, 1964).

THE
FOOD YOGI DIET

Eating more consciously now feels like a way of being. I actually think about how my food got to my plate. That was the whole point, right? – Oprah Winfrey, 2008

Ahimsa

In the broadest use of the word, *ahimsa* refers to a lifestyle of peace, and is most popularly connected with Gandhi's civil disobedience movement of the 1930s. However, in the modern context, *ahimsa* is typically tied exclusively to diet and has been popularized by Eastern spiritual movements like the Hare Krishnas. However, somewhat ironically, these same peace-loving Eastern spiritual groups have received criticism from the vegan community for their inconsistency to practice the path of *ahimsa*. Their use of commercial dairy and its ties to the exploitation of cows is a case in point.

Since the yoga path is all about connection with our higher self and God, it follows that a food yogi would walk a path of *ahimsa*, by respecting all living beings and gearing all of their thoughts, words and deeds towards a peaceful outcome. The *ahimsa* path is much more than peaceful intention; it necessitates an awareness of the spiritual equality of all beings. This awareness naturally manifests in one's choice of food.

It is rather surprising that despite the rising interest in yoga outside of India, there has not been the same degree of enthusiasm for *ahimsa* diets. In fact, many yoga practitioners in the West have not made any significant change to their diet. This can only be a result of yoga teachers not recognizing the fact that *ahimsa* is a *critical* part of the yoga tradition, which begs the question: how qualified are these yoga teachers?

Traditionally, practicing non-violence includes following a vegetarian diet. In fact, many Hindu temples in India won't even allow a person to enter the temple if they eat eggs, what to speak of meat!

In *The Hatha Yoga Pradipik*, possibly the oldest surviving text on Hatha Yoga, Pancham Sinh states: "Food injurious to a yogi: bitter, sour, salty, hot, ...intoxicating liquors, fish, meat, ...etc., should not be eaten."

McVeggies

Over the years, I have talked to numerous vegans and vegetarians who are under the impression that any kind of plant-based diet is beyond reproach. I beg to differ. While a vegan lifestyle does aim to avoid all forms of animal suffering and is therefore noble, it sadly sometimes lacks a spiritual dimension, specifically, in not honoring the Divine source from which all food originates. And while a vegetarian diet is also honorable in principle, practitioners are sometime lax in their adherence to the moral principles upon which vegetarianism is founded. This moral disconnect can be seen in the example of the "junk-food vegetarians", or "McVeggies," as they are euphemistically labeled. Such well-meaning people are really not much different than regular junk-food addicts who focus solely on the taste of food with little consideration for the quality of the ingredients or the intentions invested in the food. Indeed, like regular McDonald's customers, "McVeggies" often give little thought as to how the food is prepared, as long as they apparently contain no animal ingredients. And yet these same people with mock all "non-vegetarian" diets like fanatical religious zealots.

The irony of this "holy-than-thou" attitude was crystal clear during the McDonald's French fries scandal of 2001. The company publically acknowledged that the "100% vegetable oil" used in making their fries actually contained animal-derived flavorings, much to the chagrin of millions of "pious"

Hindus, vegetarians and vegans who frequented McDonald's thinking that they were maintaining their vows by avoiding the burgers. The New York Times[175] reported:

> When the fast-food chain announced with great fanfare that it was switching from beef fat to "100% vegetable oil" to cook its French fries, Mr. Sharma joined the legions of Hindu Americans and vegetarians who began venturing into McDonald's to nibble what they believed were vegetarian fries. Mr. Sharma's teenage son even took a job at McDonald's last year, and drawn by the generous employee discount, the Sharma family consumed countless bags of fries.

> So Mr. Sharma said he was horrified when he opened his India West newspaper in April and read, "Where's the Beef? It's in Your French Fries." He and other American Hindus were outraged to learn that McDonald's French fries are seasoned in the factory with beef flavoring before they are sent to the restaurants to be cooked in vegetable oil.

The bottom line is: it is foolish to place implicit faith in global conglomerates like McDonald's, whose principle agenda is to make profit and increase the share price for their investors and not to cater to vegan or vegetarian consumers. Vegetarian, vegan or not, we should all be concerned with what we put in our mouths. Why trust a corporate clown?

Eating the Way Nature Intended

As a person incorporates more raw fruits and vegetables into their diet, it appears this disconnect is remedied. My personal experience has shown that the more live fruits and vegetables people eat, the more sensitive, intuitive and respectful of

---

[175] *For Hindus and Vegetarians, Surprise in McDonald's Fries,* © New York Times, May 20, 2001 by Laurie Goodstein.

Nature they become. As we eat closer to the way Nature intended we become more in tune with the world around us. It is not uncommon for raw-food vegans therefore to honor the sun, Nature, or Divinity as part of their dietary regimen. Celebrity raw-food chef Chad Sarno believes doing so helps one "walk in truth":

> Preparing food with a deep connection to the Earth allows our channel to open that much more. When we bring this truth and balance into the kitchen, because the kitchen is the heart of the home, it ripples throughout all we do, feel and think. Passion is fully expressing ourselves through our work. When the fire of passion ignites inside of us, work transforms now into purpose and we are ready to walk in truth.[176]

Let me clarify, though, that, despite the overwhelming evidence supporting a raw, plant-based diet, everyone has different needs and no one diet will suit all. It is ludicrous to suggest otherwise, considering the array of human circumstances, body types, and opportunities (or lack thereof) that one may be faced with. However, in most situations, one has free choice and an adequate variety of high quality, non-violent foods to choose from, including those of the wild variety. As a rule, I believe that it is absolutely possible for everyone to eat mostly raw fruits and vegetables. For some, this might mean only 51% of their diet, while others may fully transition to 100% raw. The number is for you to decide. I once tried a 100% raw vegan diet for 2 years, and despite the expert guidance around me, I found it didn't work, and quite frankly, was damaging to my health. I now subsists on a vegan diet that is about 80% raw, however, if I am find ahimsa dairy I will gladly accept that too.

I would never endorse a diet of animal flesh, nor one that in some way compromised another conscious form of life. As

---

[176] Chad Sarno http://www.rawchef.com/

a matter of survival, however, there are times when consuming such things may be necessary. However, with the plethora of healthy food choices now available to the modern consumer, there is no justification for taking the life of another conscious, living being.

The power of prasadam

The debate over meat eating vs. vegetarian, vegan vs. vegetarian, or vegan vs. raw vegan can go on *ad infinitum*, but one diet that no one can argue with is the *food yogi diet* – a diet consisting of the purest (*ahimsa*) food in its most natural form that has been prepared with love, offered with love, served with love and then honored in a loving and highly appreciative consciousness. The *food yogi* diet accelerates one's spiritual ascension by infusing the gifts of Mother Nature with an attitude of gratitude and loving intention in order to raise one's consciousness to the absolute highest level. Such pure food is called *prasadam*[177] (mercy) in the Vedic tradition.

The *Vedas* state that such a *food yogi* diet, or a diet consisting only of *prasadam*, cannot only purify consciousness, it can literally wipe the karmic slate clean of many lifetimes! In fact, it is stated that simply by consuming such *prasadam* one time, a person can transcend this mortal world at the time of death and never reincarnate again!

For example, the Buddhist *Mahanirvana Tantra* states:

> O Devi, such pure food is not easily obtained by even great demigods. Is so potent that it can purify one's soul even if served by a dog-eater, or if taken from the mouth of a dog.[178]

> O greatest of the Devas, words cannot describe the boon of eating prasadam. Without doubt, partaking of such holy

---

[177] Pronounced: Prashardom.
[178] Verse 84.

food even one time can free the greatest of sinners of all their past bad karma. [179]

The mortal who eats prasadam *acquires as much merit obtained by one who has bathed and donated alms at thirty-five million holy places.* [180]

Indeed, the benefits of eating prasadam *cannot be described by ten million tongues and a billion mouths.* [181]

These guarantees of the *Mahanirvana Tantra* are astonishing to say the least, but they are certainly not exclusive. The *Vedas* are filled with similar statements and stories pertaining to the glory of *prasadam*.

For example the Bhagavat Purana states:

One should distribute Vishnu prasada to everyone, including the poor man, the blind man, the non-devotee and non brahmana. Knowing that Lord Vishnu is very pleased when everyone is sumptuously fed with Vishnu prasada, the performer of yajna should then take prasada with his friends and relatives. [182]

How a dog achieved liberation

Sivananda Sena, a prominent *Gaudiya Vaisnava* who lived in India during the 16th century, praised the power of *prasadam* when he narrated the story of a street dog that accompanied him and his colleagues on a pilgrimage.

Every year Sivananda would sponsor a party of two hundred pilgrims from Bengal to the holy city of Jagannath Puri to attend the annual Ratha Yatra[183] festival, some 200 miles away.

---

[179] Verses 85-86.

[180] Verse 87.

[181] Verse 89.

[182] *Bhagavat Purana* verse 8.16.56.

[183] Annual Hindu festival observed by hundreds of millions of people. The festival is based on worship of Lord Jagannath (Krishna).

One year a stray dog decided to join the group, so Sivananda arranged for his personal cooks to provide cooked rice for the dog; he even paid for the dog's fare to cross the Ganges river with them. However, when the dog disappeared one day, in a fit of anxiety, he sent the entire group to search for him. Their search was unsuccessful, but upon arriving in Puri, to their amazement, they found the great saint Sri Chaitanya feeding coconut pulp to the dog and petitioning him to praise the Lord. Remarkably, the dog began uttering the holy name. The next day, the dog disappeared again, but this time everyone understood it had attained liberation.

In his commentary on this story, Srila Prabhupada explains that, "although performed without knowledge or education [eating *prasadam* and praising God], even an animal went back to Godhead.[184]"

Prasadam can change the heart

A more contemporary example of the power of *prasadam* to transform consciousness is the one I heard first-hand from Food for Life (FFL) volunteers serving in the war-torn region of Sukhumi, Georgia in 1993.

The volunteers had been serving hot porridge and apple cider tea to needy residents in Sukhumi throughout the battle with neighboring Abkhazia. During that time, colleagues of theirs had served *prasadam* halava (sweet semolina pudding) to a major in the Abkhazian army. Unbeknown to them, this simple act of kindness would save their lives when the Abkhazians seized control of Sukhumi and went door-to-door killing Georgians on sight. Abkhazian soldiers came across the Food for Life house situated in a suburb of Sukhumi and demanded the volunteers step outside and reveal their country of origin. Most of the volunteers were Russians, and since Russia had been siding with the Georgian army the

---

[184] *Chaitanya Charitamrita Antya Lila* 1.32.

situation looked hopeless. Worse still, the leader of the group, Mayuradvaja Das, was Georgian!

However, with the courage of a lion, Mayuradvaja began explaining to the soldiers what their group had been doing for the last two years and how they had remained neutral and provided help for both sides of the conflict. The soldiers were impressed; however, orders were orders and they knew they could not take a risk, so with guns cocked they prepared to shoot. Without hesitation, Mayuradvaja spoke firmly and with earnest, "Please understand the situation here. We have a spiritual agenda and our purpose is to respect everyone. We are students of the Vedic culture of India and we believe that man is more than a physical body and is spiritual by nature." The soldiers were taken aback by his bravado and allowed him to continue. "You and I are not these bodies but are the consciousness that animates them," he explained. The soldiers hesitated, seeming to appreciate the wise words of the Georgian. "This sounds interesting," one of the soldiers responded, "but we have orders." The youngest volunteer, 15-year-old Sergey, spoke up, "I was born in Russia, but I don't consider Russia my Mother country. We all come from a higher plane of existence. These bodies are just vehicles for the soul. Please believe that we are not your enemies," he pleaded.

The atmosphere was tense with anxiety. Some volunteers cried while others prayed expectantly, hoping against hope for some kind of miracle. Mayuradvaja stood strong in his commitment to protect his men, knowing that they had acted honorably and deserved respect. He presented argument after argument to convince the soldiers not to kill the volunteers, as they had done to everyone else in the neighborhood. Considering the intensity of the circumstances, it was already a miracle that he and the others had been able to delay an inevitable massacre.

But then suddenly, as if a ray of sunshine had pierced the dark clouds that hovered overhead, the aforementioned major passed by the house and recognized that the "captives" were part of the Food for Life organization. He immediately called to the soldiers to lay down their weapons. "These boys are ok. Leave them be," he ordered.

With their hearts still pounding, the volunteers felt they had just died and come back to life. The major approached the boys and told them of his "halava experience" and offered to help them leave the city safely. *Prasadam* had simultaneously saved their lives and imbued them with irrevocable faith. They would never forget this experience.

Prisoners don't want to leave

In 2007, the *Bangalore Mirror* reported how prisoners in a state jail did not want to leave because of prasadam!

Ninemsn.com: 21 June, 2007, Bangalore, India ~ Inmates at a prison in southern India are eating so well that many are reluctant to leave while other convicted criminals are trying to move in, a newspaper said Thursday.

The Parappana Agrahara prison in Bangalore is crowded with 4700 inmates, more than twice its capacity, because small-time criminals are refusing to apply for bail, according to the Bangalore Mirror.

Juvenile offenders are also overstating their age to qualify as adults and enter the facility, the newspaper added.

The reason is the healthy food [prasadam] served by ISKCON, or the International Society for Krishna Consciousness, a Hindu evangelist organization, said the paper, whose reporters visited the facility.

ISKCON, commonly known as the Hare Krishna movement, started serving its pure-vegetarian fare in the jail on May 21 under contract from the prisons department.

Lunch and dinner typically include piping hot rice, two vegetables and a spicy lentil dish called sambar and buttermilk. A dessert is added on festival days and national holidays like Independence Day, and also once a week.

"When we are getting tasty, nutritious food three times a day here, why should we go out and commit crimes," said prisoner Raja Reddy, who has been arrested 20 times in 30 years for theft, robbery and burglary.

"Our going out of the prison will only benefit pawnbrokers who purchase stolen items at a throwaway price from us, advocates who fleece us to fight our case and the police who collect bribes," Reddy was quoted as saying.

Sraddha Ceremony

The ancient tradition of *Sraddha* is a Hindu ritual that a son performs to pay homage to his 'ancestors' and involves offering vegetarian foods to the God, Vishnu and then placing the sanctified food (*prasadam*) before pictures of his departed forefathers. It is believed that the act of offering *prasadam* to the forefathers is enough to release them from any hellish or ghostly condition they may be in.

Conceptually, *Sraddha* is a way for children to express heartfelt gratitude towards their parents and ancestors, and pray for their peace. It also considered a "day of remembrance" and is performed for both the father and mother separately, on the days they became deceased. It is also performed on the anniversary of the death, or collectively, during the *Pitru Paksha* or *Sraddha paksha* (Fortnight of ancestors), just before *Sharad Navaratri*[185] in autumn.

Vedic scholar Srila Prabhupada explains:

> *According to the rules and regulations of fruitive activities, there is a need to offer periodical food and water to the forefathers of the family. This offering is performed by worship of Viṣṇu, because eating the remnants of food offered to Viṣṇu can deliver one from all kinds of sinful*

---

[185] *Navratri* is a festival dedicated to the worship of a Hindu deity *Shakti* and is celebrated at the onset of winter (September–October in India). The word *Navaratri* literally means nine nights in Sanskrit; *nava* meaning nine and *ratri* meaning nights. During these nine nights and ten days, nine forms of Shakti or Devi are worshiped.

actions. Sometimes the forefathers may be suffering from various types of sinful reactions, and sometimes some of them cannot even acquire a gross material body and are forced to remain in subtle bodies as ghosts. Thus, when remnants of prasadam food are offered to forefathers by descendants, the forefathers are released from ghostly or other kinds of miserable life. Such help rendered to forefathers is a family tradition, and those who are not in devotional life are required to perform such rituals[186].

The Vedic tradition of *Putra* denotes that the son has a responsibility to deliver the father from any hellish condition after death. The Sanksrit word, *Putra* derives its meaning from the belief that there is a hell called *Put*, and so one who delivers (*tra*) someone from that hell is known as a *Putra*.

Sraddha is made up of two words, *Sat*: truth and *Adhar*: basis. So it literally means any act that is performed with sincerity and firm faith (*Sraddha*).

In practice, the person who performs *Sraddha* invites Brahmanas (priests) to the ceremony and imagines they are his or her parent. A fire ritual (*homa*[187]) is performed and then sumptuous food served. The son treats the brahmanas with all due respect and finally serves them "*pinda pradana*," balls made of rice that have been previously offered in prayer to Visnu and then given as sanctified food offerings to the forefathers (*Pitris*). The son then gives a donation of money to the brahmanas.

---

[186] *Bhagavad-gita* Verse: 1.41 purport

[187] Sanskrit word similar to the word *yajna* which refers to any ritual in which making offerings into a consecrated fire is the primary action. Homas are an important religious practice in Hinduism, Buddhism, Japanese Vajrayana and Jainism. A *homa* involves the kindling and consecration of the sacrificial fire on an altar made of brick, stone or copper, built specifically for the occasion and fuelled by dung, wood, and/or dried coconut shell; the invocation of one or more divinities; and, the making of offerings (whether real or visualized) to them with the fire as via media, amid the recitation of prescribed mantras.

Since *Sradhha* is one of the most important and noble "*Samskaras*[188]" that the Hindu sages have envisaged, it is imperative that the performer of the ritual understands what they are doing. Only then will the true intent of the ritual be fulfilled, and not succumb to a meaningless mechanical exercise of social convention.

The Sradhha period

During the *Sraddha* period new crops in India and Nepal are harvested and offered as a mark of respect and gratitude before other festivals are celebrated.

Crows are also considered ancestors in Hinduism and during *Sraddha* the practice of offering food to crows is still in vogue. Indeed, feeding crows is a daily ritual in the morning hours for the people of India's southern city of Chennai. The scavenger bird is considered a VIP for South Indians. The Vedic culture of hospitality clearly dictates that all food must be first offered to lower beings before being consumed by humans. After food is ritualistically offered to God, a sample is first offered to the crow.

The shrill calls of Indian maidens has its roots in the beckoning of crows to eat such food offering. It is believed the practice offered the subjugated women a chance to exercise their vocal chords. A discerning ear can even differentiate classical melodies. Mothers sometimes cajole newborns to eat by showing them the crow pecking at the food.

January is festival time for crows and a lavish spread is laid out for the birds during the sun worship festival of *Kanum Pongal*. Women of the family place different kinds of colored rice, cooked vegetables, banana and sweetened rice pudding on a plantain leaf and invite the crows to enjoy the feast. Prayers are also offered in the hope that the brother-sister ties

---

[188] Rites of passage, accomplishment, embellishment, or consecration.

may remain forever strong, just like in the family of crows. Here again we see an example of the uniting powers of food and how central it is to the culture.

EVERYTHING WE DO

Spiritual life begins with the tongue. – Srila Prabhupada

The *Vedas* state that by offering all our actions in the service of God we become purified by the fire of devotion. The example is given of an iron rod. In its natural state iron is cold and hard, and yet when consumed by fire it takes on all the qualities of fire and becomes in essence one with fire.

According to *Padma Purana,*[189] since our senses are imperfect, it is impossible to fully comprehend the magnificence of the Supreme, much the same as it would be foolish to expect an insect to understand the functioning of government, or someone with cataracts to have 20/20 vision. However, just because someone has cataracts, we should not conclude that they will *never* be able to see perfectly. At present we may not be able to conceive of God's form, but once the "cataracts" of materialistic consciousness are removed, and our senses fine-tuned to the spiritual paradigm we *will* be able to see. This cleansing of the senses begins with the tongue, and specifically through the act of offering food. The *Padma Purana* states:

> No one can understand the transcendental nature of the name, form, quality, and pastimes of Sri Krishna through his materially contaminated senses. Only when one becomes spiritually saturated by transcendental service to the Lord are the transcendental names, forms, qualities, and pastimes of the Lord revealed to him.[190]

---

[189] One of the major eighteen *Puranas*, a Hindu religious text, is divided into five parts.

[190] *Padma Purana.*

The *Bhagavad-gita* declares that one who lovingly offers his food to God, according to scriptural guidelines, is freed from all sinful reactions:

> *The devotees of the Lord are released from all kinds of sins because they eat food which is offered first for sacrifice. Others, who prepare food for personal sense enjoyment, verily eat only sin.*[191].

According to the great Law book of the *Vedas*, the *Manu Samhita*, those people who perform five pious acts[192] can counter any karma resulting from unintentional killing of microscopic amoebas during the preparation of meals; insects killed while using fire and boiling water; as well as those harmed while sweeping dirt from the house.

Since there is also killing in the harvesting of vegetables, in pursuance of these teachings, temples all throughout India perform elaborate vegetarian food offerings and then distribute the sanctified food (*prasadam*) for benefit of pilgrims.

In the Jewish tradition, spiritual practice on the simplest level is known as *avodah*, the work humans do for God. The act of *avodah* can be applied to anything if done with loving intention, as the *Kitzur Shulchan Aruch*, a nineteenth-century summary of Jewish law states:

> *(Proverb 3:6) This means to know God in all "ways" you fulfill your bodily needs, and to do them for the sake of God's name. For example, eating, drinking, walking, sitting, lying down, standing up, having sex, conversation— all the needs of your body can be for the service (avodah) of your Creator, or something that leads to it.*

---

[191] *Bhagavad-gita As It is* (Verse 3.13).

[192] The five pious acts are scriptural study, offering food to God, homage to the ancestors, feeding of animals, and welcoming and feeding unexpected guests.

How do I become a Prasadarian?

If a food yogi diet consists of eating only *prasadam*, how do we become *prasadarians*? The good news is that no prior qualification is necessary. Essentially, all that is required is sincerity of purpose. Anyone can take their existing pure food diet and raise it to the highest level of gastronomy through the process of adapting the following 10 Prasadarian Principles for higher consciousness.

1. Sincerity
2. Purity
3. Conscientiousness
4. Gratitude
5. Selflessness
6. Nurturing
7. Respect
8. Acceptance (receiving love)
9. Humility
10. Devotion

1. Sincerity

Sincerity is a very rare thing in this modern world. Too often people cut corners, compromise standards and opt for efficiency over quality. The expansion of fast food companies around the world is one obvious example – hundreds of millions of people in countries like China and India buy into the bogus marketing of these highly efficient American chains at the cost of their culture, health and the environment.

Despite their slick advertising campaigns, there is absolutely no sincerity in these corporate giants. The bottom line is profit. They will do whatever it takes to increase the share price for their investors, even if that means serving their customers genetically modified ingredients, or labeling a product as containing "natural flavoring" to appeal to vegetarians (even though the ingredients are derived from animal sources), or claiming to be a "green" company just because they participate in recycling (even though they

225

deforest ancient rainforests to provide grazing land for animals to be slaughtered for burger meat). Don't be fooled by these bogus and insincere corporations and their "greenwashing" tactics. Be sincere in your own life to seek the best for your family, the planet and yourself. Sincerity is the foundation of the Prasadarian lifestyle.

A Prasadarian is one who heeds the call to seek quality over everything else. Prasadarians spend the time to acquire and prepare the most pure ingredients. They are sincere in their efforts and do not compromise standards for anything.

Being sincere simply means to be genuinely concerned, consistent, and sensitive. So dare to be different from the masses, and always choose the path of sincerity.

2. Purity

Purity is the greatest force in the universe – the light that destroys all darkness. With purity everything is reconciled, cleansed and energized; without purity everything is eventually destroyed, decayed or lost. There simply cannot be any compromise on this principle.

When you opt for purity, you make a clear statement to the world that you value your family, the planet and yourself. Your constitutional nature is that of a pure spirit soul, so it is as natural to seek purity as it is for water to seek the deepest point. Allow your consciousness to go deep and see the essence of your very being. Do not compromise purity for glamour and hype.

In a practical sense, purity must guide every decision you make, especially when it comes to food preparation. Your kitchen therefore should be spotless at all times, and a special place in your home reserved for sanctifying your meals. When you purchase produce, select only the purest ingredients; abandon the miserly mentality of pinching pennies, and embrace the abundant mentality of offering only the best quality food. It may require smart money management and buying in bulk, but do whatever it takes to maintain a high standard of purity. Another consideration is to subscribe to CSA programs or to purchase your produce at local farmer's markets. Even better is to grow your own food.

3. Conscientiousness

Being conscientious simply means to be meticulous or careful about all that you do. To be conscientious is to live always in the moment and to maintain focus every step of the way. This constant focus is essential to the Prasadarian way of life, because it forms the very foundation from which all conscious and meaningful decisions are made. When you live in the moment, you embrace your eternal nature as a spiritual being and transcend the limiting bonds of time and space that are characteristic of this material world.

By being conscious from moment to moment, you will learn to enjoy and appreciate what you are and what you have now and will stop hankering and lamenting for things you cannot change.

Similarly, when we are conscientious about how we acquire and prepare food, it translates into powerful and enriching experiences for those we serve. Zen Buddhist Master, Thich Nhat Hanh, in his book on mindful eating, *Savor*, says, "When we water the seeds of forgiveness, acceptance, and happiness in the people we love, we are giving them very healthy food for their consciousness. But if we constantly water the seeds of hatred, craving, and anger in our loved ones, we are poisoning them."

4. Gratitude

Gratitude is the art of being thankful for all that has happened, is happening now, and will happen to you in the future. This naturally includes the blessings you receive in the form of food and water. Thankfulness must flow throughout your life. When you begin to practice gratitude, at first it may seem forced, but over time it will become a natural part of your expression. It is an innate quality of the spirit to be loving and thankful.

If appreciation and thankfulness are not part of your usual expression, it is time to change. You can start by listing all the things in your life that you are thankful for. Take that list and read it every day out loud, adding to it as more reasons for gratitude become apparent. Take this attitude into your workplace and in public, and seek every opportunity you can find to tell someone how much you appreciate them, no matter how insignificant their actions are. You will be pleasantly surprised how happy this will make you, simply because the happiness you generate from your acts of appreciation will reflect back tenfold and nurture your own spirit. This principle applies even more so when you use food as the medium to express your gratitude, because the consumed food will penetrate deep and dramatically affect consciousness. I remember when I was a young monk I would always carry freshly baked cookies to give away when visiting people. I developed such a reputation that over time, people would light up just by seeing me. Try it and see.

5. Selflessness

To be selfless does not denote losing self; rather, it means to put others' happiness first, as you would in any true, loving relationship. The most pure example of this quality is the natural love a mother expresses to her child; it is selfless in nature and very pure. The same can be said of the cow and bullock - throughout their life, the cow selflessly gives her milk, while the bullock serves the needs of the farmer by using its strong body to till the field. Therefore, in India the cow is worshipped as a mother, and the bull as a father. Sadly, even in death, these placid animals continue to selflessly serve mankind by offering the remains of their bodies in the form of meat products and leather. The modern exploitation of the cow and bull is the grossest display of ingratitude and selfishness on the planet today.

When it comes to food, to be selfless simply means to

serve others first or see to the full satisfaction of your guest's palate above your own. It is this kind of selflessness that raises one's consciousness to the highest levels of purity and satisfaction. In the Vedic culture of hospitality, making sure no one else in the village was hungry was a prerequisite to sitting down to your own meal. Being selfless with food enriches the heart and cultivates within one a strong sense of abundance, thus attracting even more food to be shared and enjoyed.

The example of King Rantideva is just one example. Following in that mood, I remember one time while on pilgrimage to a holy place[193] in India I decided to take a Rantideva[194] vow for one month for purification. The vow required that I refrain from eating or drinking anything until everyone else in the community had eaten and were totally satisfied. In the spirit of renunciation I also decided I would serve everyone else in the community their meal first and would only eat whatever remained in the serving containers. An important aspect of taking a vow is while observing them you are not to tell anyone. It must be done privately, less the benefits of the austerity be lost through a sense of pride.

With a sense of optimism and excitement I embraced the vow with full conviction and was able to complete it successfully. To my surprise, I never once felt deprived, nor did I feel powerless. On the contrary, I felt empowered and joyful. Indeed the austerity seemed to make me glow and I could feel myself getting stronger day by day, and by the grace of God, there was always just enough food remaining in the containers to satisfy my hunger.

---

[193] The holy town of Vrindavan is considered by many to be the most sacred land in India.

[194] A great Indian king of the Vedic era who took a vow to only eat after all others had been satisfied. *Bhagavat Purana* 9.21.2-15.

6. Nurturing

We are all nurturers by nature. We nurture our children, our partners and our own bodies all the time. To nurture simply means to serve with care or to nourish. True nourishment can only come from using the best quality ingredients and saturating them with the best loving attitude. When we tend to our own gardens, we also nurture and infuse the food we grow with loving intention. Such nurturing will dynamically affect the yield at harvest time, and you can be sure it will be noticeable. To be a nurturer is to serve with unconditional love and to genuinely enjoy seeing other living beings flourish and succeed. To nurture is to relish the growth and joy of another, to be happy for their happiness and, conversely, unhappy when we witness their sadness.

Modern capitalism feeds off the act of exploiting people and resources for personal gain. It is a profit-driven system and therefore if in order to realize profits, something must die or be inconvenienced, so be it. On the contrary, we find that the world's great spiritual traditions promote the idea of selfless service to others without any motivation for personal gain. Similar to the previous quality, to nurture is to love through sincerity of action.

7. Respect

To respect is to esteem someone or something. In terms of food, respect must begin at the point of gathering the seeds to grow the food. To take that a step further, we must respect the very source of our food, the sun. Some of the greatest cultures in history were worshipers of the sun. In fact, some scholars believe Christianity was founded upon sun worship.

Without the sun, nothing would exist. Respect, therefore, should begin from the time you arise every morning to greet the sun, continue when you garden or buy your produce from the store, and expand fully into a loving fiesta of respect for every ingredient as you prepare your meal. This kind of all-inclusive respect will absolutely transform your life. It will take some effort to cultivate such constant awareness as we move through our day, but with practice it can be done.

Respect by definition requires submission or subservience to a higher power and an honoring of the interconnectedness of all things. To respect is to be fully attentive at every moment.

8. Acceptance (receiving love)

When it comes to loving exchanges involving food, it's common for people to focus entirely on the giving part of the equation, when in fact receiving is just as important. We need to learn how to receive with love as much as we give with love. There is nothing so disheartening for the giver of love than for the intended recipient, out of a sense of false humility, to deny the giver the opportunity to serve. Denying love is one of the most destructive things one person can do to another. It is imperative, therefore, to learn how to receive with love and to honor those who make the effort to serve you with love.

In terms of food, we need to lovingly accept what is offered to us in love by acknowledging that act with an appreciative heart adorned with a loving smile.

I remember times while serving guests at the ashram during our Sunday service that some people did not bother to acknowledge me or the other servers when the food was placed on their plates. Rather than thanking us, they would continue chatting with friends next to them, and would sometimes even rudely announce that we had given them too much. It surprised me then and still does today that such people would not even take the time to look us in the eye and lovingly accept the food we had so lovingly prepared for them.

Similarly, it so happens that sometimes a guest at your house may persistently refuse to take an offering of food you have prepared for them because of one reason or another. However, it is always better to accept at least a portion of the offering graciously rather than rejecting the food outright. A loving relationship by definition has to consist of an endless cycle of serving and accepting.

9. Humility

The term "humility" is derived from the Latin word *humilitas*, a noun related to the adjective *humilis*, which translates as "humble" or "low." Because the concept of humility addresses intrinsic self-worth, it is always emphasized in the realm of religious practice and ethics. Humility is a spiritual virtue unrelated to the act of humiliating or shaming, which I am not suggesting here. Sri Chaitanya Mahaprabhu, a 15th century saint, scholar and mystic from West Bengal, once stated that to achieve the highest levels of devotional love one must be:

> ...more humble than a blade of grass, more tolerant than a tree, and ready to offer all respect to others.

Humility can help you get in touch with your true self. In doing so, you have a better chance of "killing" the ego. The Sanskrit word *ahankara* literally translates as "false-ego." And it is this false ego, or identification with the gross body as self, that one has to conquer in order to express one's purest devotion. The only way to achieve this is through spiritually motivated humility and certainly not by any mundane methods as Matthew (19:24) relates:

> It is easier for a camel to go through the eye of a needle, than for a rich man to enter into the kingdom of God.

In other words, true humility cannot be bought, but must be cultivated and earned. Wisdom traditions recommend approaching the spiritual realm with a humble attitude because, without humility, the full potency of the spiritual realm remains hidden beyond the veil.

As *Proverbs*[195] states: "Before his downfall a man's heart is proud, but humility comes before honor."

10. Devotion

The quality of devotion is an innate characteristic of the soul. A quality as natural to us as liquidity is to water; or heat and light is to fire; or sweetness is to sugar. These innate qualities by definition cannot be separated from their source.

Everyone has devotion, but unfortunately many either suppress it through various layers of false ego, or mask it by misdirecting its pure nature through the acts of lust. The spirit is by nature loving and full of joy, with an unending desire to serve; the problem, however, is that contact with this gross material energy pollutes the pure devotional quality of the soul, just as a contaminated atmosphere pollutes pure rain drops as they fall through the sky, resulting in modern anomalies like "acid rain."

Because pure devotion is intrinsic to the soul, it can easily be revived through controlling of the senses and purification of the mind. Many of the Eastern spiritual traditions will recommend a path of purification before one can enter into the higher teachings of that tradition. The same applies in food yoga, wherein one should ideally cultivate the previous nine qualities before fully embarking on the art of devotion.

To be a devotee is to have a heart filled with unconditional loving devotion for the Supreme Lord and to see everyone and everything in connection to the Cause of all causes.

In all spiritual traditions humanity is encouraged to serve God with devotion in all deeds. The Deuteronomy[196] states:

> "...O Israel, what does the LORD your God ask of you but to fear the LORD your God, to walk in all his ways, to

---

195 18:12 NIV
196 10:12 NIV

love him, to serve the LORD your God with all your heart and with all your soul."

Similarly, the *Bhagavad-gita* declares that one should offer all actions in service to God:

"...all that you do, all that you eat, all that you offer and give away, as well as all austerities that you may perform, should be done as an offering unto Me."[197]

According to the Quran, without *salah*, offering prayers at a mosque or elsewhere five times daily, one cannot be successful in life. Like all the major religions, devotion is mandatory. *Salah* is intended to focus the mind on God, and is seen as a personal communication with God and the devotee who expresses gratitude in his worship.

The *Bhagavata Purana* sums up the essence of devotion this way:

The supreme occupation [dharma] for all humanity is that by which men can attain to loving devotional service unto the transcendent Lord. Such devotional service must be unmotivated and uninterrupted to completely satisfy the self.[198]

In the devotional or *bhakti* traditions of India, much emphasis is given to the quality of the devotion as expressed in practical action. For example, purity is considered an absolute must for any acts of devotion. In terms of food offerings, the purity of the ingredients; the place; the methods used in preparing the meals, and more importantly, the mental purity of the person making the offering all factor into whether the food is actually accepted by God.

The question may be raised, "How do we actually know if the food was accepted by God?" The only possible way to know that is by personal experience. If the offered food makes

---

[197] *Bhagavad-gita As It Is* (Verse 9.27).
[198] *Srimad Bhagavatam* 1.2.6.

us feel enlivened in spirit and mentally pacified, we can be sure the food was indeed "touched" by the grace of God.

How to Purify Your Meal

Having come to understand the science and philosophy behind *Food Yoga*, it is now time to learn the art of spiritualizing your food and taking your eating experience to the highest level.

The Prasadarian principles described in the previous section have prepared us for the act of offering food to God. However, before we get to the actual offering procedure, it is imperative to observe the following guidelines while preparing the offering:

- **Clean body and clean work area** – This is the most important principle: nothing impure should be offered, and this necessitates having a clean working environment, clean body and clean clothes. It is also recommended to set aside a special offering plate just for this purpose – one that is used by no one else.

- **Use only food and ingredients that are pure** – Absolutely avoid all food or ingredients that involve the killing or suffering of animals, which in most cases includes dairy products. If possible, also avoid non-organic and genetically modified foods and try to use local produce.

- **Refrain from tasting the food while preparing it** – Since the ingredients that make up your meal are to be offered in love, you should honor the gifting by not tasting anything during the preparation. This may take some getting used to, but it does make a difference. The more you can prepare the meal with an attitude of complete selflessness, the more purifying the whole experience will be for you.

The Final Stage - The Offering

Having given many talks on spiritual vegetarianism over the years, I came to understand that it was important for people to feel comfortable with the act of offering food, both within the context of their own spiritual traditions and to understand the fundamentals of why we should even consider offering food in the first place. I therefore created the *Food Offering Meditation* to guide one in the act of creating higher vibration food.

With sincerity, purity, conscientiousness, gratitude, selflessness, nurturing, respect, loving acceptance, humility and, above all, devotion, use the following meditation to purify your food before you serve it.

It is important to note that this meditation first sets the framework for the humble and devotional attitude by reminding us of our temporality and absolute dependence on the grace of higher powers.

I offer this meditation as a guideline to the final stage of the offering process. I recommended that you adjust this meditation to suit the specific tradition you are accustomed to, although I believe that the meditation as it is presented herein is universal enough to satisfy all.

FOOD OFFERING MEDITATION

I am Spirit.

I was born with no possessions.

I will leave this world with no possessions.

I am neither the permanent owner nor ultimate controller of anything in this world.

Everything that has come to me has been a gift of the Supreme.

Since food is the most basic necessity of life, I therefore offer this food with loving intention back to the Energetic Source from which it came.

In doing so, I honor the Supreme Enjoyer, Supreme Creator and the Divine Feminine.

With love and sincerity, I humbly ask:
"Please taste this food."

Note: You may complete this meditation with your favorite honoring prayer.

The Meaning of the Meditation

The following notes may help to clarify the meaning and purpose of the *Food Offering Meditation*.

I am Spirit.

Self-explanatory, but the most fundamental spiritual truth and therefore the beginning of the meditation.

I was born with no possessions.

We are born naked, nameless and with no possessions. Everything we acquire in this life is in some way or another made possible by the grace or influence of Mother Earth and our ancestors. There are no exceptions. Every single one of us is and has always been dependent on the grace of someone else.

I will leave this world with no possessions.

Despite our efforts to accumulate land, money and fame, we ultimately must give them all up at the time of death. The only thing we can take with us after death is our consciousness or sense of awareness.

I am neither the permanent owner nor ultimate controller
of anything in this world.

Everything that comes to us, either through hard work or inheritance, is only temporarily under our care. Before we were here, someone else owned the land and before them, someone else. Every one of us is simply borrowing for the time we are on this planet. Similarly, despite our apparent status in material life, no one can claim ultimate control, as even a tiny microbe within our body can cause our death.

Everything that has come to me has been a gift of the Supreme.

The first symptom of true humanity is to acknowledge the many gifts of the Supreme and to offer gratitude. Many spiritual traditions begin their appreciation by honoring the morning sun while more developed spiritual traditions conduct elaborate food offering rituals.

Since food is the most basic necessity of life, I therefore offer this food with loving intention back to the Energetic Source from which it came.

We show our love and gratitude through practical acts of kindness. Offering food back to its source is natural and right and the most fundamental act of kindness. It also reinforces the fact that God has personal form and can enjoy food as we do.

In doing so, I honor the Supreme Enjoyer, Supreme Creator and the Divine Feminine.

This part of the meditation can be very personal and private. I have provided a guideline only. To acknowledge the "Supreme Enjoyer" is to accept that all living beings strive to enjoy, and that God by definition must therefore be the greatest enjoyer. Similarly, to honor God as a "Supreme Creator" is to acknowledge a divine intelligence behind all that is. To honor the Divine Feminine is to embrace the fact that masculine and feminine or the Energy and Energetic are perfected and united in the Supreme Personality of Godhead.

With love and sincerity I humbly ask: "Please taste this food first."

The final expression must be done with the utmost humility and sincerity to be effective. You could very easily include a bonafide name of God or Goddess you are familiar with. The essential point here is to offer the food with devotion to whom it originated from. At this stage of the offering you may wish to consecrate your meditation by reciting the holy name of God.

Once a portion of the food is offered, you can combine it with the food that remains in the pots (which is also now considered *prasadam*) and then serve the meal to yourself and others.

AFTER THE OFFERING

You will eat, you will be satisfied, and you will bless YHVH, your God. – Deuteronomy 8:10

Sacred Eating

In just about every contemplative tradition, eating is regarded as a sacred act. As Jewish scholar Jay Michaelson explains in his book, *God in Your Body*, "From one perspective, consuming food is simply a necessity of the body—everyone must eat to survive. But eating can also be a deeply spiritual practice, with many layers of meaning."

Michaelson suggests that, to the ancients, eating was probably just a "mysterious, and inspired gratitude, myth, and ritual," but even today there is something "miraculous about turning lettuce into 'me', and many layers of social and ritual meaning endure even in our generally deritualized society."

I enjoyed reading Michaelson's inspired notes especially the line "turning lettuce into me." How often do we stop to think about the sacrifice of the fruit, plant or vegetable we are about to consume? The lettuce, tomato and pepper *gave their life for us*. When we consume them they essentially become us. There is no clearer expression of the oneness of all life.

Conscious Eating Exercise

Now that your food has been offered and thus purified of any negative energy it may have collected along its journey into your home, it is time to enjoy. However, it would be inconsiderate and inconsistent to do so in a hurried and disrespectful manner. Therefore, the sincerity and devotion you've cultivated in preparing and offering your food should carry forth into the eating experience as well. You could call this "conscious eating," and in contrast to the typical hasty and unconscious practices of the modern fast-food culture, the act of conscious eating has its own set of rules and guidelines.

In their book *Savor*, Thich Nhat Hanh and Dr. Lilian Cheung explain that, "mindless eating and mindless living are all too common. We are propelled by the fast pace of high tech living" to the point that the "pace of our lives is utterly harried and spinning out of control. We constantly have to respond to external stimuli and demands... And our lives suffer because of it."

Location

Select a place that is clean, quiet and free from distractions, including television, Internet and radio. Eating consciously cannot be done sitting in front of the television or a computer. There must be a designated eating area in your home that has no other purpose. If you're outside, you need to select a location that will afford you the ability to fully focus on the act of eating without distraction. Eating while standing or walking is never acceptable. In fact, according to the Ayurvedic tradition, eating while standing is an invitation to poor health.

Attentiveness

To fully experience the transformative power of *prasadam*, you need to give your undivided attention to eating it, without thinking of anything else, and be still. Therefore, do not eat while doing anything else, and that includes talking on a cell phone. Make eating an exclusive exercise as you would with any meditation. Be focused.

Meditative attitude

Srila Bhaktivinoda Thakura, a prominent spiritual teacher among the Gaudiya Vaisnavas of Bengal, wrote a prayer

(*Prasada Sevaya*[199]) to be recited before partaking of *prasadam* as a way to focus one's attention and remain in a humble and meditative state of mind while eating. Much like the *Food Offering Invocation*, the prayer sets a framework for the mind before the actual praising begins.

In the spirit of making these esoteric teachings more tangible and non-sectarian I have edited the prayer as follows:

> *O Lord! This material body is a lump of ignorance, and the senses are a network of paths leading to death. Somehow or other we have fallen into the ocean of material sense enjoyment, and of all the senses the tongue is the most voracious and uncontrollable. It is very difficult to conquer the tongue in this world, but You, our divine Mother and Father, have been very kind to us. You have provided this nice* prasadam *to help us master the tongue; therefore let us take this* prasadam *to our full satisfaction while glorifying Your Lordships with loving gratitude.*

As you can see, the prayer is a little more supplicating than your typical "Grace". The essential message being conveyed here is that as souls burdened by this physical body and controlled by the ravaging senses led by the tongue, it behooves us to acknowledge the grace of blessed food and to honor it accordingly.

The following suggestions are offered as guidelines for the actual eating process. Incorporate them as much as you can in accord with the time, place and circumstance you find yourself in.

Sit upright

With your back as straight as possible, sit comfortably on a chair, mat or clean grassy area. It is important to be upright so

---

[199] The original prayer actually mentions specific names of God according to the Vaisnava (Hindu) tradition. However, I have removed them for the sake of simplicity and to focus the reader on the principle of gratitude.

that the abdominal muscles are relaxed and your breathing is in no way restricted. All seated meditation postures aim at one thing: holding the back upright without strain or slouching so that energy can run freely up and down the spine. The fundamental factor that affects this upright posture is the tilt of the sacrum and pelvis. When you sink back in a chair so that the lower spine rounds, the pelvis tilts back. When you sit up straight, you are bringing the pelvis to a vertical alignment or a slight forward tilt. This alignment is what you want for seated meditation. The placement of the upper body takes care of itself if the pelvis is properly adjusted.

Regulate your breath

Start breathing normally, but pay special attention to the timing and regularity of your breath. You don't want a quick pace, which can result from anxiousness or an unfocused mind that is thinking of something unrelated and thus not living in the moment. You want a relaxed and steady breathing pattern, which is conducive to creating the mental stability required for this exercise and will generate good *qi*, which is critical for good digestion.

Breathing is sort of a sibling to Qi – almost like twins, but not entirely identical. The air that flows through our lungs at each breath has many similarities to the Qi flow, but it is essentially different. The same applies to oxygen; the substance that breathing transports to the blood and the blood distributes to all of the body is just like Qi. Still, they are different. They are similar enough, though, for intentional and correct breathing exercises to get your Qi flowing.

Good breathing is a blessing, so delightful and stimulating that it literally inspires. Indeed the word "inspire" (from the Latin *inspirare*), means to breathe, or more precisely, to breathe in. So take a deep breath and feel your soul soar.

When you inhale you receive, and when you exhale you give. That is the rhythm of life. One is impossible without the other. Inhaling and exhaling are opposites that are forever linked, similar to *yin* and *yang* in classical Chinese cosmology.

When we breathe intentionally, we often become aware of how much this activity affects the way we think and feel. A conscious interaction with breath can help us cultivate a greater awareness of energy in general. The same applies to being more conscious in our energy exchange with others.

If you have ever studied meditation or yoga, you know that breathing consciously is much more revitalizing. It is the same with vital energy. The more you become conscious of your natural give and take of vital energy, the more profound your perception of energy will become, and the healthier you will be.

Relax the stomach

As your breathing becomes steady and relaxed, make a conscious effort to relax your stomach by visualizing it as soft and jelly-like. Allow your breath to take over; with every incoming breath, visualize the air as pure white energy entering your lungs and then moving down to expand your stomach, and with every outgoing breath, see your stomach withdraw and all your anxiety and tension drain out into the universe.

The object of your mindfulness here is not just about becoming aware of your breath, but to unite the body and mind as one. This disconnect between mind and body is the source of many weight problems, explains Thich Nhat Hanh:

> [M]any people eat without feeling hunger, or eat beyond the point of fullness, either because the food looks good to them and they crave it or because they are trying to soothe their difficult emotions.[200]

By nurturing the oneness of body and mind, and by listening to our body, "we are able to restore our wholeness ...

---

[200] *Savor*, Thich Nhat Hanh, p 72

and as body and mind become one, we need only to calm our body in order to calm our mind," he says.

Observation

Take a moment to appreciate the beauty of the food before you. Note its color, texture, and unique character. Often we barely look at our food before shoving into our mouths. You will never do that again, but will always take a moment to carefully observe the food before you. Smile at your food, and thank the person who served it to you.

Taste and smell

Now that you are relaxed, have blocked out all external distractions, and are fully focused on the food before you, it is time to focus on the senses of taste and smell. These two senses are intimately tied together. If you cannot smell properly, it will affect how things taste. Similarly, sometimes a smell is so powerful you can taste it.

Before you begin eating, tell yourself that in a few moments you are going to smell and taste everything as if these senses were completely new. All your other senses are going to be on hold while taste and smell become your main focus for sensation.

Before you take a bite, first appreciate the smell of the food. Inhale deeply and let the smell of the food inspire your appetite to the point that you're salivating.

Your first bite

Now, with a mood of great respect, take the first bite of your food, and as the morsel enters your mouth, carefully note its initial feel and flavor. Then, as you chew and move the food around in your mouth, continue focusing on the changing flavors and texture of the food as it breaks down and mixes with the digestive juices inside your mouth, all the while keeping a mood of respect and gratitude flowing through your mind.

Note how the different parts of your tongue have receptors for different tastes. The tip is sensitive to sweet, while the back of your tongue has receptors for bitter. You taste salty foods with the taste buds on the side of your tongue. Be aware of this as you chew, closing your eyes so you can immerse yourself in the experience.

Chew slowly

According to the *Ayurveda*, grains should be chewed 32 times before swallowing. Doing this for the first time can be a tiring experience, but it will teach you to thoroughly break down your food, thus aiding digestion and maximizing the nutritional benefits of the food. I suggest that the first time you do this you close your eyes and focus all your attention on the experience. If counting your chews doesn't appeal to you, have a friend assist you by asking them to tell you when one minute has elapsed.

A good friend of mine, Melissa Klein[201] of *sun Compass Wellness* in Washington DC, introduced me to the technique of sounding a small bell while eating. As I closed my eyes and chewed my food, she would gently remind me when a minute had passed, and thus when I could take another bite. The exercise helped me to maximize every single bite, and I must say it also helped my digestion tremendously.

Horace Fletcher (aka "the great masticator") was a great proponent of the healthful benefits of thoroughly chewing food. Author of *In Defense of Food*, Michael Pollan comments: "At fifty [Fletcher] could bound up and down the Washington Monument's 898 steps without pausing to catch his breath - while existing on a daily regimen of only 45 well chewed grams of protein."

---

[201] http://www.suncompass.net/

Swallowing

As you swallow the food, imagine a pure white ball of energy entering your body, slowly passing down your throat and moving towards your stomach where it will very soon surcharge and enliven every cell of your body. The food is becoming your new body! You truly are what you eat, so make the eating experience a meaningful and beautiful one, and prosper.

Paying Attention

The more attention you give to the eating experience, the greater chance your digestion will be strong and efficient, because you will not only be tuning into the sensual joy of the food, but also listening to your body and acting accordingly. By eating slowly, you give the stomach a chance to catch up to the pre-digestion taking place in your mouth. It takes only minutes for food to reach the stomach; the feeling of "fullness," however, is not determined by the filling of the stomach, but rather by an increase in blood sugar. For a meal that includes fat, carbohydrates, and proteins, this signal to the brain can take about 20 minutes. But if the meal is high in protein or high in fat, it may take 40 minutes to an hour for that "fullness" feeling to kick in, because the stomach has to first digest the proteins into useable carbohydrates before delivering them to the bloodstream. Only then does the blood sugar rise and signal "full" to the brain.

The ramifications of inattentive eating are obvious: the stomach gets so packed that digestion is hampered, leading to poor assimilation of the food, feelings of low energy and reaching for yet more food. Much of the obesity epidemic in the world is a result of inattentive eating habits. A good rule of thumb to avoid overeating is to keep in mind that the stomach requires water and air to properly digest food. The Ayurveda suggests that the ratio should be 50% solid food, 25% water and 25% air. To understand this better, imagine packing your kitchen processor with solid food to the top of the container and trying to run it. How effective would the processing be? Now, take some of that food out and add a little water and leave some space for air and just see how much better the "digestion" will be.

In his *Imitation of Christ*, Thomas a Kempis explained:

> When the belly is full to bursting with food and drink, debauchery knocks at the door.

Francine Prose, in her book, *Gluttony, the 7 Deadly Sins*, says, "...we cannot be mindful of God or our final end or even of our human nature or moral responsibilities when, carried away by gluttony, we are behaving like the animal that came to symbolize the sin - that is to say, the pig."

Slow Down

A practical way to avoid over-eating is to either take smaller bites or to put your utensils down between bites, thus forcing yourself to give full attention to the food that is in your mouth at that time and resisting the temptation to keep adding more.

With a quiet mind and contemplative spirit, a true spiritual transformation can take place. As the prophet Isaiah says, "Pay attention to Me, and you will eat that which is good, and enjoy the delights of your soul." [202]

A Healthy Eating Regimen

Naked Lunch – a frozen moment when everyone sees what is on the end of every fork. – William S. Burroughs

The first rule of a healthy eating regimen is to never eat when you're angry, depressed, bored, or otherwise emotionally unstable. Nor should you eat immediately after any physical exertion.

---

[202] Isaiah 55:2

It is a good practice to bathe, or at least wash your hands, face and feet, before you begin to eat.

When feasible, eat with your hands (without the use of utensils), so that your skin can send temperature and texture cues to your brain. It is said that digestion begins with sight and feel of the food and not by mastication alone.

If at all possible, face east, the direction of the sun, the earth's source of heat and fire. Eat alone or with people you know and respect. Listening to soft music and lighting incense will pleasantly stimulate your other senses and enrich the experience.

Remember that satiation of hunger is not determined by how much you eat; rather, even a small amount of food presented to you lovingly will satisfy your spirit, whereas large helpings of food from a fast-food restaurant may temporarily fill your stomach but will leave your mind and spirit unsatisfied and most likely agitated.

Allow only those who love you to prepare your meals. Cooks in India are often selected from the *brahminical* (priestly) class so that there is at least a chance that some spiritually uplifting vibrations may be transferred into the food while cooking. It is recommended that women not cook when they are menstruating because their bodies are undergoing a cleansing process, often resulting in an agitated mind, so they should be relaxing instead.

According to the *Ayurveda*, it is best if your right nostril functions when you eat, since it increases the digestive fire. You can help to accelerate this function by lying on your left side for a few minutes before and after the meal or by closing your left nostril with the middle finger of your right hand and breathing rhythmically through your right nostril for a few minutes.

Another important principle learned from India's Vedic culture is to feed someone else before you begin. In India, after food has been prepared, a five-fold offering is traditionally made to the sacred fire, a cow, a crow, a dog, and another human being, who might be a child, a beggar, or anyone else outside one's own family. This is how one thanks Mother Nature in a practical sense - by feeding some of Her children in gratitude to Her. It is also another way of controlling *ahankara* (egoism) and acknowledging that all food is intended not for mere self-gratification, but for the greater good of all beings. Feed anyone - a pet, a plant, a neighbor, or a stranger - so that you can experience a little of Nature's joy - the joy that a mother feels when she feeds her children and watches them grow and develop in consequence.

In the next chapter we look at India's spiritual hospitality culture and how the concept of offering and sharing *prasadam* was an integral part of that culture's success.

INDIA'S VEDIC CULTURE OF HOSPITALITY

No one within ten miles of our temple should go hungry.
– Srila Prabhupada

No One Should Go Hungry

Is anybody hungry? Please come to my home, where my wife has prepared a meal. We have enough to feed 20 hungry men. She has prepared the finest rice, curry, and puris (fried bread). I will not take my meal until I know that every man, woman, and child is fed.

Such selfless gestures of hospitality were common in the village life of ancient India. The religious householders of the Vedic times saw themselves as providers for all living beings, including the animals. No creature was allowed to go without food during the pinnacle of Vedic civilization. This is the fertile ground in which the seeds of Food for Life's philosophy were sown.

Within the Vedic hospitality tradition there are six loving exchanges, as explained in this verse by a 15th century Vedic scholar, Rupa Goswami:[203]

Offering gifts in charity, accepting charitable gifts, revealing one's mind in confidence, inquiring confidentially, accepting prasada and offering prasada are the six symptoms of love shared by one person and another. (Verse 4)

---

[203] Rupa Goswami (1489-1564) was an Indian devotional teacher (*guru*), poet, and philosopher from the Gaudiya Vaisnava tradition of Hinduism.

We can see that in ordinary social activities, these six types of dealings between two respected friends are absolutely necessary. For example, it is very common for business to be conducted over dinner. One man will inquire from the other how he should conduct his business, and often gifts are exchanged. Whenever there are dealings of love and respect, these six actions can be found.

The Meaning of Hospitality

According to the Oxford Dictionary, hospitality is "a friendly and generous reception of guests or strangers." To be hospitable, therefore, means to care and show respect for another being. It is a sincere expression of appreciation, love, and humility. A person whose heart is filled with gratitude, magnanimity, and spirituality is naturally hospitable.

It's important to note that hospitality is not the same as entertaining, which is, unfortunately, the more common approach today. When we entertain, we put all of our effort into the event – the appearance of the home, the rich, high-calorie/low-nutrient food and refreshments, and seating and table settings. We judge the success or failure of the event by such unimportant details as whether or not the napkins matched the décor or the ice ran out. In contrast, hospitality focuses on the comfort and wellbeing of guests; the desire to freely share one's home; the nutritious, life-giving food that is prepared; and, above all, the people.

In her book, *Gluttony, the 7 Deadly Sins*, Francine Prose notes:

> *In the Greco Roman tradition, feasting along with drinking was the social cement that enforced the values of the citizen and kept the state together. Good feasts and bad feasts are reoccurring motifs at the center of the Odyssey, where it is made very clear that the worth of the host depends upon the generosity of his table.*

Some hosts put so much energy into preparations for

entertaining that they have little left for their guests. By the time the guests leave, the host is exhausted. Hospitality, on the other hand, is physically and spiritually refreshing and nourishing. Simply put, entertaining is fueled by pride, while spiritual hospitality as espoused in the Vedic tradition arises out of true humility and wisdom.

Spiritual hospitality does not distinguish based on species, race, caste, creed, or color; these differences are meaningless from a spiritual perspective. Rather, spiritual hospitality welcomes all with a loving embrace. For an example of profound hospitality, one need not look any further than the example of King Rantideva of India's Vedic tradition.

The Story of King Rantideva

Rantideva is glorified, not only in human society but also in the society of the demigods (devas), for his exemplary tolerance, compassion, and selflessness.

Rantideva never endeavored to earn anything. He would enjoy whatever he received by providence, but when guests came he would give them everything. Thus he, along with the members of his family, endured considerable suffering. Indeed, he and his family members shivered for want of food and water, yet Rantideva always remained sober. Once, after fasting for forty-eight days, in the morning Rantideva received some water and some foodstuffs made with milk and ghee, but when he and his family were about to eat, a brahmana (priest) guest arrived.

Because Rantideva perceived the presence of the Supreme Godhead everywhere and in every living entity, he received the guest with faith and respect and gave him a share of the food. The brahmana guest ate his share and then went away.

Thereafter, having divided the remaining food with his relatives, Rantideva was just about to eat his own share when a sudra (field worker) guest arrived. Seeing the sudra in relationship with the Supreme Personality of Godhead, King Rantideva gave him also a share of the food.

When the sudra went away, another guest arrived, surrounded by dogs, and said, "O King, I and my company of dogs are very hungry. Please give us something to eat."

With great respect, King Rantideva offered the balance of the food to the dogs and the master of the dogs, who had come as guests. The King offered them all respect and obeisance.

Thereafter, only the drinking water remained, and there was only enough to satisfy one person, but when the King was just about to drink it, a chandala (outcaste) appeared and said, "O King, although I am low born, kindly give me some drinking water."

Aggrieved at hearing the pitiable words of the poor fatigued chandala, Maharaja Rantideva spoke the following words:

I do not pray to the Supreme Personality of Godhead for the eight perfections of mystic yoga, nor for salvation from repeated birth and death. I want only to stay among all the living entities and suffer all distresses on their behalf, so that they may be freed from suffering.

By offering my water to maintain the life of this poor chandala, who is struggling to live, I have been freed from all hunger, thirst, fatigue, trembling of the body, moroseness, distress, lamentation and illusion.

Having spoken thus, and although on the verge of death because of thirst, King Rantideva gave his own portion of water to the chandala without hesitation, for the King was naturally very kind and sober.

Suddenly, out of thin air, great demigods (devas) like Lord Brahma and Lord Siva, who can satisfy all materially ambitious men by giving them the rewards they desire, then *manifested their own identities before King Rantideva, for it was they who had presented themselves as the brahmana, sudra, chandala and so on. (Bhagavat Purana 9.21.2-15)* [204]

The great demigods had tested the King for his level of tolerance and compassion and the great King succeeded and thus received their blessings.

Another beautiful example of selfless sacrifice can be seen in the story of King Yuddhisthira's[205] *Asvamedha* ritual[206] performed around 3000 BC. At the time, it had been considered the greatest religious ceremony in history. However, when the assembly was glorifying King Yudhisthira a strange looking mongoose arrived in the ceremonial arena. Half of his body was golden and the other half normal. Suddenly, the mongoose started to roll on the sacrificial altar and then, to the great astonishment of all, he stood up and spoke in a human voice: "I don't agree that this is the greatest sacrifice," he announced to the assembled priests. The people asked, "why are you declaring this?" to which the mongoose replied, "a long time ago there was a great famine and people were starving everywhere. There was a *brahmana*[207] family who didn't have any food for many days, so one day, the *brahmana* went out to beg food grains. After some time, he came home and his wife prepared a meal. As they were just about to eat, there was a knock on the door. The *brahmana* opened the door and saw that it was a travelling mendicant, so he invited

---

[204] © Bhaktivedanta Book Trust.

[205] From the Hindu epic *Mahabharata*, *Yudhisthira* (Sanskrit: "steady in war"). He was the eldest son of King Pandu and Queen Kunti. He was the king and leader of the Pandava side in the *Kurukshetra* war mentioned in the *Bhagavad-gita*. For his piety, he was also known as *Dharmaraja* ("king of dharma").

[207] *Brahmana* (Sanskrit) – a member of the highest Hindu caste, that of the priesthood.

him in. The mendicant said he was very hungry, so without hesitation, the head of the family asked the man to sit down. "Some food has just been prepared, so please eat," said the *Brahmana*. The pious *brahmana* offered his share of the meal and the visiting mendicant ate heartily. However, he said that he was still hungry, so the *brahmana*'s wife then offered her share. And yet he was still hungry, so the son offered his share. Finally, the daughter offered her share and only then did the mendicant feel satisfied. That night the *brahmana* and his family died of starvation, but upon dying, a golden chariot descended from the spiritual realm to liberate them."

According to the mongoose, they died the most honorable deaths, and he was so impressed by their selflessness and humility, that he considered the home to be the most sanctified place on the planet. With great humility he started to roll on the floor and the food grains that were lying on the ground touched his body. That half of his body that the food grains touched mysteriously became golden. He continued, "Since then, whenever I hear of some sacrifice being performed, I go there and I roll on that ground, with the anticipation that the other half of my body will become golden. But it hasn't happened yet, and it didn't happen here. That is why I am emphatically declaring that the mighty King *did not* perform the greatest religious ceremony."

The mongoose's touching story serves to illustrate that grandness is not necessarily synonymous with virtue. We all have the capacity to touch another person's heart through the simplest acts of devotion and humility, mixed with selfless sacrifice. It is not the packaging that counts, but the loving intention that resides within. That, in essence, is what the Vedic culture of hospitality is all about and it perfectly captures the meaning of food yoga.

FOOD FOR LIFE

With roots in ancient Indian culture, Food for Life is a modern-day revival of the Vedic custom of hospitality, which was based on the understanding that all beings are equal.

In 1974, shocked and saddened at the sight of children in a poor village fighting with street dogs over scraps of food, A.C. Bhaktivedanta Srila Prabhupada, told his yoga students: "No one within ten miles of a temple should go hungry . . . I want you to immediately begin serving food." Heading Srila Prabhupada's instructions, Krishna devotees were inspired to establish a global network of free food kitchens, cafés, vans, and mobile services. The humanitarian project, then known as ISKCON Food Relief, quickly expanded to the West, with daily delivery routes in many large cities around the world under the new banner of "Hare Krishna Food for Life."

From feeding the poor and homeless on a local level, Food for Life emerged as a competent emergency food relief service, serving hot vegetarian meals to survivors of natural and man-made disasters. In 1995, a formal headquarters, Food for Life Global, was established in Washington, DC to manage and support the worldwide expansion.

Food for Life volunteers have been involved in some of the most demanding emergency relief efforts in modern history, including

- The war in Sarajevo, Bosnia-Herzegovina in 1992
- The earthquake that devastated Latur, India in 1993
- The war in Grozny, Chechnya in 1994
- Earthquake in Latur, India 1998
- Earthquake in Gujarat, India 2001
- The tsunami disaster in Sri Lanka and India, 2004 - 2005
- Hurricane Katrina and Hurricane Rita in 2005
- The Haiti earthquake in 2010

- Pakistan earthquake in 2010
- Tsunami relief in Japan in 2011.

Today, Food for Life is the world's largest plant-based food relief organization, with thousands of volunteers in over 50 countries. The non-profit has served over one billion free meals since 1974.

Mission

Food for Life's mission is to *bring about peace and prosperity in the world through the liberal distribution of pure plant-based meals prepared with loving intention.*

As simplistic as this statement may appear on the surface, the fact is that a plant-based diet can not only feed more people, dollar for dollar, but also directly and indirectly improve the quality of life – and therefore the prosperity of the earth's entire eco-system.

It's important to understand that Food for Life is more than a food relief organization and that its aim is not simply to solve world hunger. Rather, Food for Life believes that food in its purest form is the best medium for loving exchange and, therefore, a cure-all for the disharmony that plagues our planet. In essence, therefore, Food for Life is an organization focused on creating peace and prosperity by using the medium of pure food.

Pure food, by definition, means purity on all levels and in every stage of production. Such food is a blessing to anyone who comes in contact with it. This is the philosophy of food that Food for Life projects pride themselves on and encourages others to adopt. Indeed, pure food is not the monopoly of any particular religious or spiritual tradition, but rather is a human birthright and should be made available to all sincere seekers.

Aims and Objectives

Food for Life Global projects span the globe, and while each project has its own unique local strategy, all *bona fide* Food for

Life Global projects embrace the following aims and objectives as their guideline:

- **Welfare:** To provide pure plant-based meals to the disadvantaged, the malnourished, and victims of disaster (natural or man-made), wherever there is a need in the world.
- **Education:** To establish Food for Life education centers throughout the world. These centers will provide free or low-cost meals, counseling, yoga classes, and living skills training.
- **Youth Development:** To establish Rural Academies for Youth (Food for Life R.A.Y. of Hope), in which young people between the ages of 16 and 25 are trained in sustainable agriculture, yoga, cow protection and personal wellness.
- **Non-Violence:** To reduce the number of animals slaughtered for food by sharing with as many people as possible the higher taste of plant-based meals.
- **Hospitality:** To revive the ancient Vedic culture of hospitality, and to teach by example that there is spiritual equality among all beings.

"Uniting the World Through Pure Food"

One may wonder why an international food relief organization has a slogan – *Uniting the world through pure food* – that essentially talks more of peace than hunger relief. The answer is simple: Food for Life Global is not only a food relief organization, but also a social change organization that uses pure food and all things related to the production of pure food as its principle medium.

This is why the programs are so diverse and include partners such as *Working Villages International* (www.workingvillages.org), arguably the world's leading example of a self-reliant eco-village, and other project partners like the Sandipani Muni school for the poor in northern India (www.fflvrindavan.org), and the sustainable education services

261

of *SANTEE* in West Virginia, US.

Indeed, Food for Life Global projects represent a complete solution for world peace, prosperity and health. We believe that, because food speaks all languages, the purest food – food that is grown, prepared and served with pure intention – can nourish not only the body, but the mind and soul as well. It is the kind of food that can uplift the spirit and illuminate the consciousness; pure food will unite people while healing past hurts.

Pure food, by nature, is also good for the planet, as it is grown without chemical fertilizers and herbicides and with full consideration for the long-term health of the soil, the protection of natural wildlife, and the environment as a whole. Rather than contribute to global warming as the intensive factory farms of the meat industry do, pure food cultivation nurtures and actually improves the planet over time.

All food prepared and distributed by Food for Life is first energetically purified with loving intention and then sanctified, a practice rooted in Hindu tradition that is similar to the *Food Offering Meditation* discussed earlier. Sharing food has been a custom in many cultures since the beginning of civilization, however, and people of all faiths are familiar with the spiritual practices of thanksgiving and offering to God the first of the earth's yield. The meals provided by Food for Life are prepared and served in this manner to nourish both body and soul.

Spiritual Equality

Fundamental to the Food for Life program is the belief that all beings are spiritually equal. Without this understanding, none of Food for Life's projects could prosper, nor could the program embrace such a diverse, yet interdependent set of programs. For example, by promoting a plant-based diet, Food for Life not only seeks to reduce the damage caused by factory farming of livestock, but also to demonstrate that animals should be respected and loved as much as any human child. Similarly, the forests and rivers that help to grow the food are living with as much or more importance as any human entities. After all, the earth was here long before humans began populating it.

Seeing the spiritual equality of all living beings is essential to cultivating the compassion and purity to evolve beyond the shackles of our material bodies and to spiritualizing our eating, for those who eat the rotting flesh of animals are nothing but cemeteries on legs. Or, as George Bernard Shaw put it:

> A man of my spiritual intensity does not eat corpses.

Various religious traditions have a great deal to say about spiritual equality, as seen in these passages from some of the world's holy books.

The Bible:

> Have we not all one father? Has not one God created us? (Judaism and Christianity[208])

The Bhagavad-gita:

> The humble sage, by virtue of true knowledge, sees with equal vision a priest, a cow, an elephant, a dog and a dog eater. (Hindu[209])

The Qur'an:

> Have you not seen how that God sends down water from the sky, and therewith we bring forth with it fruits of diverse hues? And in the mountains are streaks white and red, of diverse hues, and pitch black.

---

[208] Judaism and Christianity. Bible, Malachi 2.10.
[209] Bhagavad-gita As It Is (Verse 5.18).

Men, too, and beasts and cattle are of diverse colors. Even so only those of His servants who have understanding fear God. (Islam).[210]

Bahia Faith:

Light is good in whatever lamp it is burning. A rose is beautiful in whatever garden it may bloom. A star has the same radiance if it shines from the east of the west....all are members of one family – children of one Heavenly Father. Humanity may be likened unto the multi-colored flowers of one garden. There is unity in diversity. Each sets off and enhances the other's beauty. (Abdul Baha)

The Sutta Nipata:

So what of all these titles, names, and races? They are mere worldly conventions. (Buddhism[211])

With a hint of sarcasm, Gandhi[212] once said: "I believe in equality for everyone, except reporters and photographers."

If you look at the outer dress of humans or any other species, you can easily see the differences. To see the spiritual essence and equality of all beings, however, requires contemplation and a higher sense of knowing. Such vision, according to the Gita, is only afforded to those who are both pure and humble. Spiritual knowledge must be earned.

Universal Respect for All

Atithi Narayana, another concept derived from the ancient Vedic culture, is also a central belief of the Food for Life program, instilled by Srila Prabhupada as the program's fundamental purpose. Atithi means unscheduled or unannounced, and Narayana is one of the many names of Vishnu (God). Atithi Narayana therefore means that the

---

[210] Qur'an 35.27-28.
[211] Buddhism. Sutta Nipata 648.
[212] Mahatma Gandhi (1869–1948).

unannounced visitor to one's home should be respected like God.

It's hard to imagine such hospitality in Western countries today, with so much crime, distrust, and fear. In ancient Vedic times, however, it was common for the householders to call out into the streets for those who were hungry to come and be fed. Indeed, it was a common practice to call out three times, and only after all others had been satisfied did the householder himself enjoy his meal.

John Robbins, author of the bestselling *Diet for a New America*, writes, "The existence of so much hunger in the world is a reality we cannot deny. It is a reality that challenges us deeply: it asks us to become more fully human." From his contemporary perspective, Robbins sees finding a solution to world hunger as the responsibility of every human being on the planet:

> *When we remember those who are without food, something is awakened within us. Our own deeper hungers come to surface – our hungers to live fully, to bring our lives into alignment with our compassion, to make our lives expressions of our spirits.*

Spiritual equality, elimination of hunger, world peace...while Food for life recognizes that these are lofty ideals; the organization is founded on the principle that these ideals are attainable.

Food for Life Projects

Food for Life provides a variety of feeding programs in cities and villages around the world, with each program developed according to local need and community support.

Free and low-cost cafés

Food for Life cafés first appeared in Australia in the early 1980s, setting a standard that other non-profit feeding programs are still trying to emulate. Designed to serve the homeless, single mothers, and the elderly, the cafés offered an all-you-can-eat menu for a nominal donation. Thanks to generous contributions from local businesses and individuals, those who couldn't pay were never turned away.

Menus change daily. A typical menu consists of Indian curries, hot breads, basmati rice, chutney, semolina pudding and a drink; on other days, an Italian meal might be served. In Australia, the Food for Life services are legendary, having saved the day for tens of millions of people over the years.

Delivery services

But what about the elderly, the sick, and the homebound? No one needs pure, wholesome food more than they do, and yet it is harder for them to come by it. Food for Life volunteers address this need by delivering food to those who can't travel to a FFL restaurant or distribution point.

Food for Life Meals on Wheels began delivering fresh vegan meals to the elderly and homebound in Australia in the 1980s. In areas where funding and staffing such a program is impractical, Food for Life has partnered with existing community feeding programs to provide a vegan alternative one day each week.

Food for Life's largest and most successful food delivery initiative, however, is its participation in the Indian government's Midday Meal program, which was established to protect children from classroom hunger, increase school enrolment and attendance, and improve socialization among children of all castes.

Since 2001, Food for Life Global affiliates, ISKCON Relief Foundation (IFR) through their *Food for Life Annamrita* project and the Akshaya Patra Foundation have operated ultra-modern centralized kitchens all over India through a public-private partnership. More than 2 million meals are delivered to schools in sealed, heat-retaining containers just before the lunch break every day! These projects feature some of the best menus in India's school meal program, with tasty vegetable curries, rice, vegetables, and hot breads. See: www.annamrita.org & www.akshayapatra.org

Emergency Food Relief

When natural or man-made disasters strike anywhere in the world, Food for Life volunteers spring into action, preparing and serving hot, nutritious meals to survivors. Over the years, Food for Life has responded at the scene of dozens of earthquakes, floods, hurricanes, and wars, including the following.

Grozny, Chechnya (1994–1996)

Taking leave from their corporate jobs and coming from as far away as Moscow, Food for Life volunteers endured great personal hardship to operate the city's only food program during the 20-month conflict in Chechnya. In his column in *The New York Times*,[213] journalist Michael Specter chronicled the remarkable job done by volunteers in the midst of deplorable conditions.

Their makeshift mobile "kitchen" was a 10-year-old discarded ambulance. The buildings in which they lived and worked were shell-damaged and surrounded by debris, with "no windows and few doors." Yet in the midst of these primitive and dangerous conditions, Food for Life volunteers prepared and served more than 2 million vegetarian meals and baked "what some people consider the best bread in Grozny," according to Specter. In describing the local community's response to the volunteers, Specter wrote:

> Here, they have a reputation like the one Mother Teresa has in Calcutta: it's not hard finding people to swear they are saints. In a city full of lies, greed, and corruption, the Krishna's deliver the goods.

---

[213] c. 1995 N.Y. Times News Service.

Asian Tsunami (2005)

In what was arguably the most successful emergency relief effort in the history of Food for Life, volunteers from more than 15 countries converged on Sri Lanka, India, and Malaysia to provide hundreds of thousands of hot vegan meals to stranded survivors of the catastrophic 2005 tsunami.

Food for Life volunteers in South India were the first responders, bringing hot vegan meals to survivors literally hours after the first waves hit shore. Just a few days later, volunteers from the US, Croatia, Australia, Poland, Hungry, Sweden, Italy, England, India, and Mauritius converged on Colombo to begin feeding programs around the island.

Over the ensuing months, volunteers set up temporary cooking facilities in schools and shelters managed by the Sri Lankan army. The villagers offered to assist in cutting vegetables, while Food for Life cooks toiled over large pots cooking over firewood. The facilities were as basic as one might imagine in a disaster zone, but no one complained. Food for Life volunteers were happy to see the smiling faces of the people they served, who relished everything offered to them.

Hurricane Katrina (2005)

Once again, Food for Life was a first responder to one of the worst natural catastrophes in history, Hurricane Katrina. Soon after the hurricane passed, volunteers at the FFL farm in Carriere, Mississippi, began cooking and serving hot vegan meals to needy families in the surrounding areas of New Orleans. "Fortunately, our Food for Life kitchen was not damaged during the hurricane," explained Maharani Devi Dasi, who oversaw the preparation and distribution at the FFL emergency relief kitchen.

Soon after distribution began, Food for Life Global in Washington DC arranged for truckloads of organic produce and equipment to expand relief operations. As relief efforts ramped up, FFL volunteers from Mississippi, West Virginia,

Washington DC, and Florida arrived in the Gulf Coast towns of Waveland, Biloxi, and Gulfport to distribute vegan meals to hurricane survivors.

Courageous volunteers ventured into the hardest-hit areas of the Gulf Coast, braving fields of debris, vast stretches of noxious quick mud, and desperate, delirious locals to distribute freshly cooked vegan meals. Despite reports of people being held up at gunpoint to feed gas-hungry SUVs and pickups, FFL volunteers journeyed to Gulfport and Biloxi to bring hot meals of red beans and rice, chapattis, and lemonade to the starving residents.

Since 2005, hundreds of thousands of meals have been served by Food for Life volunteers to Gulf Coast residents.

Children and Education

An educated child grows to become an integral part of the social fabric; their learning and skills shape the nation. Sadly, however, children are the most helpless victims in the face of poverty, hunger, and illness. Through its education and support programs, Food for Life creates hope for the future by helping children grow into strong and healthy adults with the knowledge and skills to build a better world. Two of those programs are described here.

Gokulam Orphanage

Food for Life's premiere orphanage is Gokulam-Bhaktivedanta Children's Home. Located minutes from Colombo, Sri Lanka, Gokulam is a safe haven for destitute and orphaned children that serves as a benchmark for service organization around the country.

Gokulam helps the children achieve the self-confidence, determination, and integrity to grow into productive and successful world citizens through a holistic approach that includes:

- **Physical Health** – The children are served three full, balanced, vegetarian meals every day, prepared according to strict nutritional and hygiene guidelines.

Physical activities and regular exercise, along with the watchful care of medical professionals, also promote good health.

- **Spiritual Health** – The children learn to see each other and all humans as brothers and sisters, regardless of background, ethnicity, or history. Gokulam's non-sectarian approach teaches universal spiritual values such as love, faith, unity, and respect for all religions.

- **Emotional Health** – The children who find refuge at Gokulam either have no family or have seen their families devastated by civil war, poverty, and natural disasters. Here they receive unconditional love and acceptance in a warm and welcoming family atmosphere.

- **Education** – The well-rounded, progressive education offered at Gokulam includes technical/vocational training, recreation, and the arts, as well as academics. Courses are taught in three languages and include both theoretical and experiential learning opportunities tailored to individual needs.

For more information on the orphanage, visit www.gokulam.org

Food for Life Sandipani School

At the Sandipani Muni School in Vrindavan, Food for Life offers free education, meals, and medical care for 1500 of India's poorest children. The program provides school uniforms and seasonally appropriate clothing to every child, and students receive the tools and confidence they will need to become productive adult members of society. The Sandipani Muni School has received numerous accolades from the Indian government.

Recognizing the relationships between hunger and other social problems like unemployment and poverty, Food for Life Vrindavan (FFLV) is engaged in programs to alleviate the root causes of these conditions. FFLV provides the poorest of the poor with basic needs and essential services, including:

- **Basic medical assistance:** Seven days a week, FFLV doctors provide free medical treatment to hundreds of mainly women and children who otherwise have no access to medical assistance.
- **Training courses for women:** Women in Vrindavan are often exploited, illiterate, poverty stricken, and living in the most unsanitary conditions. Providing women with skills that will lead to self-sufficiency is FFLV's highest priority.
- **Drilling for drinking water and constructing water tanks:** For the past five decades, the water in the villages around Vrindavan has been contaminated with water so salty even the animals couldn't drink it, and villagers were constantly ill. FFLV has brought sweet drinking water to 40,000 people in six villages, and delivery to additional villages is in progress.
- **Assistance to the elderly and the disabled:** These are the people who suffer most from the effects of extreme poverty, and widows are especially vulnerable in a society where women have virtually no rights. FFLV takes special care of the defenseless.
- **Environmental projects and education:** FFLV maintains a tree nursery and an organic farm, distributing tree saplings to villagers. FFLV has planted more than 3,000 to date in villages, schoolyards, and playgrounds, educating children about the importance of protecting and maintaining the environment.

Volunteer Diary

By now you know that Food for Life is a multifaceted organization of volunteers dedicated to *bringing peace and prosperity to the world through the liberal distribution of pure vegan food prepared with loving intention.* You also have a general overview of the kind and magnitude of food relief and welfare services FFL provides around the world. There is no better way to understand the heart of Food for Life, however, than through the eyes of a volunteer.

The following is an entry from my personal diary as I joined other volunteers in feeding the survivors of the 2005 tsunami.

Sri Lanka, January 26, 2005 – On Saturday we traveled down South to meet our food relief team in Matara. On the way we witnessed the incredible scale of the destruction, as literally hundreds of miles of coastline had been wiped out. At one point we stopped to view a train that had been hit by the wave. As I surveyed the area, I came across hundreds of personal items, including a child's shoe. The sad story was obvious.

Our team in Matara has been cooperating with the Sri Lankan military to provide hot meals to various refugee camps in the area. The people down south have a very particular taste – they love chilies, salt and loads of rice cooked a very particular way. So our team of cooks made the necessary adjustments and soon began serving thousands of meals daily. The other unique feature of the relief here was how the meals were being served. Rather then have everyone sit down or line up in front of our pots, the local soldiers and some villagers helped us to scoop the rice, dhal and vegetable curry into a plastic wrap, that was then packaged inside sheets of old newspaper.

Major General Kulatunga told me, "this is military style." I must say, it was extremely efficient under the circumstances. The meals stayed hot for a longer time while we traveled to each refugee camp to distribute them.

One of our volunteers offered Food for Life Volunteer T-shirts to anyone that would help with the cutting of vegetables and food distribution. Talk about enthusiasm! He was swarmed like a Rugby scrum as children and adults pleaded for one of our bright yellow t-shirts.

The next day, the Major General suggested we move our operations to a more needy area of the island. We had to agree; it was becoming clear now that the military had done an excellent job of providing food for these camps. Food for Life was instrumental in making sure no one went hungry during the early stages of the relief, but it was time now to move on. Our team packed up, loaded the truck with the remaining rice and vegetables and headed back to Colombo. Next stop: Batticaloa, on the far east side of the Island and one of the hardest hit areas, where we will join our other relief team.

Since the beginning days of the tsunami relief, Food for Life has been operating in the east in the main port of Trincomalee. Indeed, Food for Life was the first food relief agency to respond to the tsunami victims. Our team continues to provide much-needed food and counseling in this area, and soon another team from the south will join them in the nearby city of Batticaloa. We expect to close down both these operations in the next few months as the situation continues to normalize and transition from relief to reconstruction.

Testimonials

Nelson Mandela:

Another important building block for new democracy is the love and goodwill we show to each other. That is the spirit of Masakhane, of bringing one another together. It is also the spirit of today's festival organized by Food for Life.

Salambek Hadjiev (Former Prime Minister of Chechnya):

I pray that your FOOD FOR LIFE program will expand to bring about a peaceful world.

Arlen Specter (US Senate):

I congratulate you for your fine achievements on behalf of the homeless....FOOD FOR LIFE's success in providing housing, food, and social services has long attracted the attention of this office.

Susan Tydings Frushour (Red Cross)

Many people were in tears to see the efforts of the FFL volunteers. Many of those who received it commented that it was the best food they have had in a long time, even before the hurricane hit!

Thabo Mbeki (Deputy President of South Africa):

FOOD FOR LIFE is the real Reconstruction and Development Programme. The understanding that if I have a plate of food, let me share it with my neighbor . . . let those who are feeling sad come together with us, and together we can share this burden. This understanding should be taken from FOOD FOR LIFE and transmitted to the entire country.

Zola Dowell (OXFAM):

As one of FOOD FOR LIFE's supporters, OXFAM has witnessed firsthand the organization's activities and its ability to reach vulnerable groups in a caring and respectful manner.

Leland Montell (International Rescue Committee)

On behalf of the IRC, I would like to compliment the efforts of FOOD FOR LIFE in providing fresh fruit, vegetables, and prepared meals to some of the most vulnerable groups in Serbia.

Hayley Mills (British actress)

I am sure that in every city where there is a FOOD FOR LIFE program, the people would be very grateful for the help they give—feeding hundreds and hundreds of people, *that would otherwise cost the city a great deal. And all the support, friendship, and counseling—it's hard to put a value on something like that.*

The New York Times

"...here they [FFL volunteers] have a reputation like the one Mother Teresa has in Calcutta: it is not hard finding someone to swear they are saints."

Vegetarian Times

"... though it may not get top mention on the nightly news, FOOD FOR LIFE is among the world's most intrepid relief organizations, in at least one case delivering food to a war-torn region after the Red Cross and other agencies gave up."

Financial Express India

"In Bangalore, Jaipur and other cities, Akshaya Patra (FOOD FOR LIFE) meals are cooked in the most modern kitchens and good quality food is delivered to schools. Corporate bodies should also be involved in this process by creating public-private partnerships like Akshaya Patra." – Comments by Prime Minister Atal Bihari Vajpayee

Financial Times of London

"...while the Kremlin has been willing to spend trillions of rubles on its soldiers, only one Russian civic organization has come to Chechnya to provide emergency aid for its often homeless and sometimes starving compatriots – the Russian branch of FOOD FOR LIFE."

Police Gazette (Australia)

"The fact the police and the Food for Life organization are looking to work together ...... represents very positive policing."

Moscow Tribune

"The Food for Life cooks have established themselves as the chief emergency feeding program in war-torn Chechnya."

SACRED FOODS

According to the *Ayurveda* every food engenders an alchemical reaction (earth, water, fire, or air) upon our body when consumed. The effect will either be positive or negative, depending on our own unique bodily constitution. However, there are some foods that stand in a class of their own for their power to increase spiritual awareness and intuition, while others can apparently help foster integrity and morality!

The following fruits, vegetables, nuts and seeds have a history in sacred ritual and spiritual development. They are not only healthy for our physical body, but also nourishing to our mind and spirit and therefore should be included in your food yogi diet.

Alchemically Active Meals

You may wish to use this list as a practical guide for preparing sacred and alchemically active meals. An alchemically active meal will simultaneously work on your physical, psychological, and spiritual expressions. A perfectly designed alchemically active meal is one that is a balanced fusion of elemental forces (earth, water, fire, air), each contributing their unique elemental signature.

When planning your meals, it is important to consider not only the alchemical properties of the food, but also the physical, mental, and spiritual makeup of those who will eat the food. For example, passionate or aggressive people might do best on foods high in the Water Element to help calm them down, whereas lazy or depressed people will benefit by eating Fire Element foods to vitalize them. Similarly, worldly persons should be fed plenty of foods high in the Air Element to uplift their consciousness, while intellectuals, idealists or fanatical religious zealots would do well on a diet of Earth Element foods to ground them.

While there are numerous combinations of these elements, the principles of balancing them are relatively straightforward. The art of creating an alchemically balanced meal comes through understanding the hidden elemental signature; matching that with the qualities of the people, and applying that knowledge based on time, place and circumstance to invoke positive transformation.

A food yogi cook therefore needs to be an intuitive and insightful physiologist, psychologist, and spiritualist with a heart filled with loving intention. Keep these points in mind when preparing meals. Each food in this list has been assigned a value of one of the four archetypal elements: Earth, Water, Air, and Fire and is based on the research of renowned alchemist Dennis William Hauck. The predominance of a particular element in a food is denoted by up to three plus (+) signs, indicating the highest amount.

Almonds are the king of nuts and are sacred to the gods Thoth, Hermes, and Mercury. In the Old Testament, the almond was a symbol of watchfulness and promise due to its early flowering. In the Bible the almond is mentioned ten times, beginning with Book of Genesis 43:11, where it is described as "among the best of fruits."

Similarly, Christian symbolism often uses almond branches as a symbol of the Virgin Birth of Jesus; paintings often include almonds encircling the baby Jesus and as a symbol of Mary.

Almonds are said to foster wisdom by stimulating intuition and insight through the Third Eye Chakra.

However the wild variety of almond are bitter and deadly because the kernel produces deadly cyanide upon mechanical handling. Eating even a few dozen at one sitting can be fatal. Only the sweet domesticated almonds should be consumed.

Unlike most other nuts, almonds increase alkalinity in the body. Almonds are an excellent source of vitamin E, magnesium, manganese, copper, phosphorous, and B vitamins. A one-ounce serving has 13 grams of good unsaturated fats, just 1 gram of saturated fat, and is always cholesterol free. When compared to other nuts, almonds are the highest in protein, fiber, calcium, vitamin E, riboflavin, and niacin.

It is best to soak almonds overnight and then discard the water. The soaking removes digestive enzyme inhibitors and revitalizes the nuts. The *Ayurveda* recommends adding pre-soaked almonds to heated fresh cows milk as a brain tonic.

I add soaked raw almonds to my vegan morning smoothies. Try to use pesticide-free raw almonds. If possible, US consumers should buy direct from the farmer to avoid the pasteurization laws. Since 2007, California almonds labeled "raw" must be steam-pasteurized or chemically treated with propylene oxide. This doesn't apply to imported almonds or almonds sold from the grower directly to the consumer in small quantities. The treatment also isn't required for raw almonds sold for export outside of North America. [Earth ++]

Amaranth is a relative of spinach and chard that was domesticated about 7000 years ago by the Aztecs who regarded it as their sacred grain. Zuni legends relate that amaranth was one of the plants brought up from the underworld at the time of their emergence.

Amaranth plants are members of an elite group of photosynthetic super-performers that are super efficient in converting soil, sunlight, and water into plant tissue.

Amaranth is higher than milk in protein, calcium, magnesium and silicon, and the United Nations FAO has found that wherever it is consumed there is no malnutrition.

Amaranth is a cooling, astringent food, beneficial to congested lungs. [Earth +++]

Anise is a calming spice. It relaxes the body and mind. Anise has been used to treat menstrual cramps. Anise seeds contain the phytoestrogen Anethole, which is 13 times sweeter than sugar and has a carminative effect on the body. Such phytoestrogens may also protect against prostate, breast, bowel, and other cancers, cardiovascular disease, brain function disorders and osteoporosis.[214]

According to plant magic traditions, placing anise seeds in a small cotton bag under your pillow will help prevent nightmares. Anise leaves are also claimed to protect a sacred space.

Anise helps cure insomnia. Aniseed tea is good for nursing mothers, as it is believed to increase milk production. The sweet-smelling tea made from star anise enhances meditation. [Air ++]

Apples are known as the Fruit of the Gods. Because of their geometric symmetry they are considered a powerful source of spiritual energy that encourages balance and harmony. The Egyptians offered apples to their highest and most powerful priests, whom they considered guardians of hidden knowledge. In Norse mythology, the goddess *Idun* provides apples to the gods that give them eternal youthfulness. In ancient Greece, the apple was considered to be sacred to Aphrodite, and to throw an apple at someone was to symbolically declare one's love; and similarly, to catch it was to symbolically show one's acceptance of that love.

Research suggests that apples may reduce the risk of colon cancer, prostate cancer and lung cancer. The fiber contained in apples reduces cholesterol by preventing reabsorption. The maxim, "an apple a day keeps the doctor away," has merit. Apples are a great source of fiber and therefore can help those suffering from constipation. [Air +++]

Apricots have been cultivated for over 5,000 years in the mountainous regions of China. Because they contain a feminine energy they are often used to lighten a person's nature. The best dried apricots come from Turkey and are dried in the sun. Apricots are rich in vitamins and minerals and therefore help strengthen the immune system. Seeds or

---

[214] *1. Albert-Puleo M (December 1980). "Fennel and anise as estrogenic agents". J Ethnopharmacol .*

kernels of the apricot grown in central Asia and around the Mediterranean are so sweet, that they may be substituted for almonds. Apricot seeds were used against tumors as early as AD 502. In England during the 17th century, apricot oil was also used against tumors, swellings, and ulcers. They are also a component in traditional Chinese medicine. It should be noted that apricots are one of the most heavily sprayed fruits and therefore you should choose only the organic varieties. [Air ++]

Barley grass juice or powder is a concentrated nutritious whole food that is easily digested by the body, and considered a *powerful psychological grounding agent* and physical energizer. It has a very strong alkalizing effect on the body. In plant magic traditions barley is used for love, healing and protection.

Barley grass powder contains very large amounts of vitamins, minerals, amino acids, enzymes and other beneficial nutrients, including high amounts of vitamin B12 (80mg per hundred grams), vitamin C (7 times more than oranges), calcium (11 times more than cows' milk), iron (5 times more than spinach) and chlorophyll.

I prefer barley grass powder for my smoothies over the more expensive spirulina. [Earth +++]

Basil (Holy Basil) also known as *Tulasi* or *Tulsi* is sacred to Hindus and is worshipped as an avatar of goddess *Lakshmi*. Water mixed with tulasi leaves is given to the dying to raise their departing souls to heaven. Tulsi, which is *Sanskrit* for "the incomparable one", was a consort of Krishna in the form of *Lakshmi*. There are two types of tulsi worshipped in Hinduism: "Rama tulsi" has light green leaves and is larger in size and "Shyama tulsi" which has dark purple leaves.

Vaishnavas traditionally use japa malas (rosary beads) made from dried tulsi stems or roots, which are an important symbol of initiation. Tulsi necklaces are considered to be auspicious for the wearer, and believed to put them under the protection of Krishna.

All forms of Basil are most powerful eaten raw. According

to herbal lore, basil has potent love properties and therefore should be used when casting love spells. Traditionally, Vaisnavas will always add tulasi leaves to food offerings made to Lord Krishna. The sacred herb soothes anger and promotes love and devotion by simulating the Heart Chakra.

All kinds of basil strengthen the immune system and is known to kill bacteria. In *Ayurveda*, tulasi is regarded as a kind of "elixir of life" and believed to promote longevity. In a study[215] in 1998, tulasi showed some promise for protection from radiation poisoning and cataracts. [Fire +]

Bay leaves are sacred to Lord Vishnu, the Maintainer of the Universe in Hindu theology. They were known as laurel leaves to the Greeks and were believed to increase psychic powers. Priestesses of Apollo chewed the leaves and inhaled their smoke to induce a psychic state of mind. Many ancient mythologies glorify the laurel tree as a symbol of honor. In plant magic traditions they are used in spells for protection, psychic powers, healing, purification, and strength.

They have many properties that make them useful for treating high blood sugar, migraine headaches, bacterial and fungal infections, and gastric ulcers. [Fire +++]

Beans were thought to contain the souls of the dead in ancient Egypt and Greece, and it was forbidden to eat or crush the plants. They were deposited with the dead in ancient Egypt. Beans promote correct decision-making and are often used in divination rituals. Azuki beans (known as the "king of beans" in Japan) are one of the most digestible varieties, as are the green mung beans from India.

Peas are a variety of sweet bean that according to feng shui promotes luck in romance and money. Some kinds of raw beans, especially red and kidney beans, contain a harmful toxin (lectin phytohaemagglutinin) that must be removed by cooking.

---

[215] *Indian Journal of Pharmacology* 30 (1): 16–20. (1998)

In many cuisines beans are cooked along with natural carminatives such as anise seeds, coriander seeds and cumin, as well as asafoetida, which reduces the flatulence that beans can create.

However, fermented beans will usually not produce most of the intestinal problems that unfermented beans will, since yeast can consume the offending sugars. Fermentation is also used to improve the nutritional value of beans. If you plan to cook your beans, soaking them overnight and then discarding the water will remove most of the complex sugar known as Raffinose, which is the main cause of flatulence from beans.

I encourage sprouting all kinds of beans to get the most nutritional value. A very effective way to sprout beans like lentils or azuki is in colanders. Soak the beans in water for about 8 hours then place in the colander. Wash twice a day. The sprouted beans can be eaten raw or cooked. Alchemically, consuming beans increases [Air +++]

Beets stimulate the Heart Chakra, inspire higher passions and represent love of beauty. They are powerful detoxifiers and when included in juices help to cleanse the liver, gall bladder and kidneys. The red roots were sacred to the Greek goddess of love, Aphrodite. The leaves and stems of beats are high in vitamin C and therefore a great addition to any salad. The Romans praised beets as an aphrodisiac. Beetroot juice has been found to improve performance in athletes, possibly because of its abundance of nitrites. The Nitric Acid that beets produce in your body open up blood vessels so that blood can surge throughout your body - to your heart, brain, and sexual organs, etc.

The juice of beets is an excellent natural red or pink food coloring. Raw foodies will just grate the beet into a salad or on a sandwich, rather than boiling it first. [Earth +++]

Broccoli is sacred to the god Jupiter, and therefore the Romans believed it increased physical strength and inspired leadership qualities. Broccoli is considered a superfood because of its amazing blend of nutrients and anti-cancer compounds. Broccoli is rich in minerals such as potassium, calcium, phosphorus, iron, zinc and sodium, and vitamins such as B1, B2, B6, E and especially ascorbic acid (vitamin C) and carotene (provitamin A). It is best eaten lightly steamed for maximum nutritional benefit, however, it can be eaten raw. I often use it as an ingredient in my pumpkin seed pâtés. Alchemically broccoli increases [Water ++]

Cacao (*Theobroma Cacao*), also known as cocoa, is not a "bean" but in fact the almond-like seeds of the cacao pod fruit. Cacao powder comes from grounding these seeds, while the white cacao butter, also called theobroma oil, is a pale-yellow, pure, edible vegetable fat extracted from the cocoa bean.

The Mayans considered chocolate beverage sacred and called cacao "Food of the Gods." In fact, cacao seeds were used by the Mayans and later by the Aztecs as currency. When the conquering Spanish came to realize the value of cacao seeds, they called them black gold (*oro negro*).

Raw, unprocessed cacao seeds raise emotional energy, heighten intuitive and psychic abilities, and induce feelings of love by stimulating the Heart Chakra. Unprocessed cacao is high in antioxidants (six times more than blueberries), and is also nature's primary source of magnesium, which happens to be the most deficient major mineral in the modern human diet. It is interesting to note that the center of the chlorophyll molecule is magnesium. According to Joel Brenner in his book, *The Emperors of Chocolate*, cacao is the most pharmacologically complex food source in the known Amazon jungle, containing an estimated 1,200 individual chemical constituents!

The base chemical in cacao, theobromine, has about a quarter of the stimulating power of its sister molecule caffeine. Unlike the hyperactive effects of caffeine, theobromine gently stimulates the central nervous system, relaxes muscles and helps dilate blood vessels.

Processed chocolate does not have the same healthful

benefits as raw cacao. The denaturing of the cacao seeds through roasting and addition of milk, excessive processed sugar, and chemicals diminish the benefits. [Fire ++]

Catnip (*Nepeta cataria*) is sacred to Bastet, the Egyptian cat goddess, and is believed to inspire happiness, calmness, and increase life force. The plant has been consumed as a tea, juice, tincture, infusion or poultice, and has also been smoked. Catnip tea encourages wonderful dreams and soothes strained nerves and helps in the relief of bloating and stomach nausea from colds and flu. According to herbal lore, Catnip is a magnet for positive energies and luck; it can also be used in love spells in conjunction with the placing of a rose quartz and red rose petals. [Water ++]

Coriander, also known as cilantro, Chinese parsley or dhania, is said to instill peace in the mind, inspire thoughtfulness and increase intelligence. It can be used as a diuretic to reduce blood pressure and ease headaches. Because heat diminishes their flavor, coriander leaves are often added to a dish just before serving. The leaves and seed contain antioxidants. Coriander is also reputed to help with the relief of anxiety and insomnia, and in holistic and traditional medicine, it is used as a carminative and digestive aid. In the *Ayurveda*, coriander is considered an herb in the mode of goodness. Interestingly, the reaction on the body is an increase in fire. [Fire ++]

Cinnamon comes from the same family as the laurel tree and is therefore thought to increase spirituality and psychic awareness by stimulating the Crown Chakra.

Cinnamon was imported to Egypt as early as 2000 BC. It was regarded as a gift fit for kings and its oil was used in Egyptian mummification rituals. The Hebrew Bible makes specific mention of the spice when Moses is commanded to use both sweet cinnamon and cassia in the holy anointing oil,[216] as well as in *Proverbs* where the lover's bed is perfumed with myrrh, aloes, and cinnamon.[217]

Ninety percent of the world's highest grade of cinnamon comes from Sri Lanka. The inferior cassia, which is thicker and darker in color, is a variation of the spice. Cinnamon is an antiseptic and painkiller and when it is burned as incense or added to foods, cinnamon not only helps to warm the body, but also raises spiritual vibration. [Fire +++]

Coconut has a long history as a food that increases chastity and purifies the body and mind. Coconut milk is sacred to the Greek goddess of wisdom (Athena). Coconuts are an essential element of rituals in Hindu tradition. The Hindu goddess of well-being and wealth, Lakshmi, is often shown holding a coconut. In Hindu wedding ceremonies, a coconut is placed over the opening of a pot, representing a womb.

Coconut water is known to be one of the most balanced electrolyte sources in nature, making it an excellent rehydration drink. It is also a powerful alkaline-producing food. The coconut tree is an extraordinary gift of nature, providing a variety of edible products – coconut water, oil, butter, cream, malai (meat), vinegar, "palm cabbage," sugar crystals, syrup and even a type of "soy sauce" when the sap is mixed with sea salt. In some parts of India, the coconut palm is known as *kalpa vriksha*, meaning, "the wish-fulfilling divine tree," although the banyan, sacred fig and *parijat* are also considered as such. Eating coconut is said to inspire tolerance, acceptance and spiritual receptivity. [Water ++]

Dandelion is sacred to the Greek lunar goddess, Hecate. It is similar to the plant, catsears ("false dandelions"), but whereas the leaves of dandelions are smooth, those of catsears are coarsely hairy. The bitter-tasting root of the dandelion is used to call forth spirits to fulfill desires. When the root is roasted and ground like coffee, the infusion not only

---

[216] Exodus 30:22-25
[217] Proverbs 7:17

increases one's psychic powers but is also said to open a doorway through which enlightened spirits can communicate. Unlike coffee bean, dandelion root is not acidic to the body.

Dandelions have been used in herbal medicine to treat infections, gall bladder, liver and urinary tract diseases. It is a good diuretic, which is probably why it is known as *pissenlit* (piss-a-bed) in modern French. The leaves contain abundant vitamins and minerals, especially vitamins A, C and K, and are good sources of calcium, potassium, iron and manganese. It is the bitterness in dandelion leaves that makes them so good for your digestion. The bitter taste stimulates secretion of the digestive fluids, including stomach acid, bile and pancreatic juices. The flowers don't look very edible, but they are good eaten straight off the plant, and are mild and slightly sweet. Eating a few dandelion flowers often relieves a headache too. Dandelion grows wild just about everywhere, but most people ignore it thinking it to be a useless weed. [Air +++]

Dates are a kind of palm fruit that have been cultivated in Africa for over 7,000 years. They were considered sacred in Babylon and Greece, and the Hebrews made syrup from them as an offering to God. Dried dates are considered fruits of the spiritual world and are symbolic of the eternal resurrection of the soul. The best varieties are the *Amir Hajj, Empress* and *Medjool* dates. Although dates represent simplicity, paradoxically, they are said to make one sexually potent and therefore a yogi seeking control of the mind and senses will minimize the use of this fruit.

In Islamic culture, dates and yogurt or milk are traditionally the first foods consumed for *Iftar* after the sun has set during Ramadan.

Dates are a very good source of dietary potassium, protein, fiber, and trace elements including boron, cobalt, copper, fluorine, magnesium, manganese, selenium, and zinc.

In India and Pakistan, North Africa, Ghana, and Côte d'Ivoire, date palms are tapped for the sweet sap, which is converted into palm sugar (known as jaggery or gur). [Air +++]

Dill was considered sacred to the Egyptian god, Horus. Both the dried plant and seeds stimulate the Sacral Chakra. Dill's dominant masculine energy stimulates sexual desire if eaten in excess. The Romans fed dill to gladiators to instill courage. Dill should be minimized by yogis wishing to follow a path of celibacy, although it can help to ease flatulence, hiccups and indigestion. Dill tea can help increase the production of breast milk. [Fire +++]

Fennel was considered sacred to the Greek god of ecstasy, Dionysus. It is one of the nine plants invoked in the pagan Anglo-Saxon *Nine Herbs Charm*, recorded in the 10th century. In Greek mythology, Prometheus used the stalk of a fennel plant to steal fire from the gods. It appears that the alchemical reaction of increased fire in the body, help to improve eyesight.

According to herbal lore, fennel will repel all evil spirits. You can hang it near windows and doorways, or carry it with you for protection.

Like saffron, fennel inspires a sense of joy. For personal use, fennel can be infused into a delicate, spiritually purifying, physically healing tea that eases nausea, relieves gas, and helps arthritic conditions. The herb is sometimes fed to cows to stimulate their milk production. [Fire +++]

Figs are one of the first plants cultivated by humans – well before the domestication of wheat, barley, and legumes. The biblical quote "each man under his own vine and fig tree"[218] has been used to denote peace and prosperity. Egyptian priests always bit into a ripe fig at the conclusion of consecration ceremonies. The Greeks considered them the ideal food. In Asia, the banyan fig tree is sacred to Buddha and is said to have its roots in heaven. Prophet Muhammad claimed: "If you say that any fruit has come from Paradise, then you must mention the fig, for indeed it is the fruit of

---

[218] *(1 Kings 4:25)*

Paradise. So eat of it, for it is a cure for piles and helps gout."[219]

Figs symbolize the rewards of meditation. The many seeds in the fig are supposed to signify unity and the universality of true understanding, knowledge, and sometimes faith. The fig trees of East Asian tradition stood for knowledge acquired by meditation.

The word "fig" actually comes from the Arabian word for testicles, though esoterically, they are thought to embody only the purest denotation of love. I recommend organic Brown Turkish and Mission figs. Nutritionally, figs are one of the highest plant sources of calcium and fiber. Figs have a laxative effect and contain many antioxidants. According to USDA, Mission figs are richest in fiber, copper, manganese, magnesium, potassium, calcium, and vitamin K. They are alkalizing to the body. [Air +++]

Hazelnuts are sacred to the German god Thor. They stimulate the Third Eye Chakra and are sometimes eaten to increase intuition prior to divination rites. The hazelnut, as well as the bark and leaves of the tree have all been used against various ailments. The tree is considered the symbol of marriage, abundance and family happiness, while the hazelnut is honored as the symbol of peace, health, wealth and power. The versatile nuts also help increase fertility. They are rich in protein, Vitamin E, minerals, dietary fibers, and contain significant amounts of Vitamin B^1 and B^6. [Earth ++]

Honey is one of the most ancient foods and was gathered even before the advent of agriculture. Honey was sacred to many gods, including the Egyptian sun god *Ra* and the Greek earth goddess, *Demeter*. Happiness and fulfillment are two qualities universally associated with the nectar.

Raw honey is the concentrated nectar of flowers that comes straight from the extractor; it is the only unheated, pure, unpasteurized, unprocessed honey. This type of honey

---

[219] *Foods of the Prophet - Qur'an 55:10-13*

contains ingredients similar to those found in fruits, which become alkaline in the digestive system. It doesn't ferment in the stomach and it can be used to counteract acid indigestion. When mixed with ginger and lemon juices, it also relieves nausea and supplies energy. Raw honey has the most nutritional value and contains amylase, an enzyme concentrated in flower pollen which helps predigest starchy foods like breads.

Raw honey can be used internally as food and externally as an antibacterial. It is a powerful antioxidant, and the Manuka brand of honey from New Zealand has powerful antibiotic properties. It is also excellent for treating colds, flu, and headaches. Unfortunately, if one wishes to follow an *ahimsa* diet, honey would generally not be included, because bees do suffer in the collection of most commercial honeys. However, there are some honeys like the tribal or wild variety that are extracted without harming the beehive. There is also a multi-flora natural honey brand in India called *Shreejee Honey that* is produced by non-violent methods.

Once when Gandhi made a reference to "innocent honey," one of his friends asked what he meant by the expression. Gandhi answered:

"Honey scientifically drawn by scientific bee-keepers. They keep the bees and make them collect honey without killing them. That is why I call it innocent or non-violent honey. That is an industry which admits of great expansion."

"But can you call it absolutely non-violent? You deprive the bee of its honey, as you deprive the calf of its milk," replied the friend.

"You are right," remarked Gandhi, "but the world is not governed entirely by logic. Life itself involves some kind of violence, and we have to choose the path of least violence. There is violence even in vegetarianism, is there not? Similarly, if I must have honey, I must be friendly to the bee and get it to yield as much honey as it will. Moreover, in the scientific bee-culture" the bee is never deprived of its honey altogether."[220] [Water +++]

Lettuce is often associated with female or lunar goddesses. Esoterically, lettuce invokes feminine energies for protection and psychic centering. Ancient Egyptians thought lettuce to be a symbol of sexual prowess and a promoter of love and childbearing in women.

Folk medicine has also claimed it as a treatment for pain, rheumatism, tension and nervousness, coughs and insanity. It contains a natural sedative called lactucarium, which relaxes the nervous system and induces sleep.

Depending on the variety, lettuce is a good source of vitamin A, vitamin K and potassium, with higher concentrations of vitamin A found in darker green lettuces. While most varieties of lettuce predominantly carry the Water element, romaine and red varieties carry more of the Air Element. [Water ++]

Mango is sacred to Buddha, and it is considered one of the most spiritually charged and elevating fruits of all. They stimulate the sacral chakra. In Hinduism, the perfectly ripe mango is often held by Lord Ganesha as a symbol of devotional perfection. Mango blossoms are also used in the worship of the goddess of learning, Mother Saraswati. In Tamil Nadu, the mango is considered, along with banana and jackfruit, as one of the three royal fruits.

Mango trees have an extraordinary lifespan and can bear fruit after 300 years! These trees have very deep roots and the flowers are wonderfully fragrant. Mangoes therefore help cultivate stability and a high level of individuation. Mango fruit pulp is high in vitamins A and C. [Air +++]

Milk from protected cows that is unpasteurized and unhomogenized is considered "liquid religion" amongst Hindus and is therefore one of the most *sattvic* of foods.

---

[220] *Collected Works/Volume 65/Discussion On Swadeshi* (28th September 1934)

Krishna, the original form of Lord Visnu, is a divine cowherd boy.

According to the *Ayurveda,* such pure milk is considered a complete food because it has the qualities of *ojas*[221] – the essence of all *dhatus* and is thus equal to nectar.

By definition, *pure* cow milk is milk that is given with love (hand milked) by cows that are protected and never raised for slaughter. Because the cow represents the Divine Feminine, her milk has the ability to inspire divine consciousness and emit subtle vibrations of the divine nurturing energy (*Shakti*). As a result, according to the *Ayurveda,* when we drink a protected cow's milk, the cells in our body get charged with *sattvica* (goodness) and the peace giving qualities present in the milk. [Water +++]

Millet comes in some 7000 varieties and is one of the seven sacred grains. Wild millet was part of the Balkan diet as far back as 6000 BC, and Japanese farmers grew it around 5000 BC. Before the recent agricultural revolution, the staple diet for Asians was millet with minimal use of rice or wheat. Millet is disease resistant unlike cereals like rice and wheat, so they do not require any pesticide. Unlike most grains, millet is alkaline-forming, so it may help to neutralize acidic conditions in the body, such as arthritis and rheumatism. [Earth +++]

Mustard was sacred to Aesclepius, the Greek god of healing. It increases alertness and opens higher mental channels, allowing one to become aware of hidden threats or evil influences. Hindus believed that eating mustard seeds would allow them to travel out of their bodies and gain awareness of other worlds.

This plant is used in phytoremediation to remove heavy metals, such as lead, from the soil in hazardous waste sites

---

[221] *Ojas* is a Sanskrit word that literally means "vigor." *Ojas* also means light and, in the *Ayurveda,* it is considered the essential energy of the body – equated with the "fluid of life," and is the essence of all the *dhatus.*

because it has a higher tolerance for these substances and stores the heavy metals in its cells.

Mustard greens grow wild in many forests around the world. Like the seeds, the leaves are also very high in the Fire Element. [Fire +++]

Nutmeg is the dried fruit of the tropical nutmeg tree that is believed to promote health and fidelity and attract good fortune. Nutmegs were put inside Egyptian mummies and often carried as lucky charms in ancient Europe. Nutmeg tea eases rheumatism and pain in the nerves. The dried outer shell of the nutmeg is ground into a spice called mace, which is sacred to the Greek god, Hermes.

For the ancient Arabs, nutmeg was a primary treatment for nausea, shortness of breath and even skin disorders. Nutmeg aroma has also been found to stimulate the Sacral Chakra of women and is therefore considered an aphrodisiac for them. The Hindus embraced the spice for its sensual properties as a stimulant in raising body heat and sweetening breath. Nutmeg has traditionally been highly prized by Chinese women as an aphrodisiac.

Nutmeg is also said to inspire lucid dreaming and to help with dream recall. Nutmeg has been used for its effectiveness to treat nervous complaints and to promote sound sleep. [Fire ++]

Olives are said to promote spiritual aspirations and build integrity. They were sacred to the Egyptian supreme solar god, Aten. The olive branch is a universally heralded symbol of abundance, glory and peace. They were used as emblems of benediction and purification and ritually offered to deities and powerful figures.

Olive oil has long been considered sacred; it was used to anoint kings and athletes in ancient Greece and was burnt in the sacred lamps of temples as well as the "eternal flame" of the original Olympic games. Victors in these games were crowned with its leaves.

The Prophet Mohamed is reported to have said: "Take oil

of olive and massage with it – it is a blessed tree."[222]

When eaten whole, olives increase sexual potency and fertility and hence should be eaten sparingly by food yogis practicing celibacy. Virgin olive oil should not be heated and is best used in salads or on foods after they have been cooked. [Air ++]

Oranges are derived from a mystical fruit called the citron and are alkalizing to the body. It was known to the ancient Chinese and in Sumeria became sacred to Enlil, the god over earth and air. Citrons were used in ancient religious ceremonies for their invigorating fragrance. All varieties of oranges provide purifying energy for both body and mind. In some Wiccan rituals, orange juice is drunk instead of wine, and orange peel tea is said to keep one from getting drunk or muddleheaded. The vitamin C in citrus fruits raises the brain's level of norepinephrine, which increases energy while reducing irritability. Oranges stimulate the sacral chakra.

Although not as juicy or delicious as the flesh, the peel is edible and has higher contents of vitamin C and more fiber. It also contains citral, an aldehyde that antagonizes the action of vitamin A. Oranges are a good and practical source of Vitamin C, although broccoli, kiwi and parsley contain more than double the amount.

It is best to blend oranges into a fruit smoothie, rather than juice them, as many of the valuable nutrients and fiber is present in the pulp. [Fire ++]

Pomegranate is sacred to Persephone and Ceres, gods of growth and fertility. Ancient Egyptians regarded the pomegranate as a symbol of prosperity and ambition. In the Ancient Greek mythology, the pomegranate was also known as the "fruit of the dead." In some artistic depictions, the pomegranate is found in the hand of Mary, mother of Jesus. In Judaism, it is said that Solomon designed his coronet based on the pomegranate's "crown" (calyx). Some Jewish

---

[222] *Sunan al-Darimi*, 69:103.

scholars believe that the pomegranate was the "forbidden fruit" in the Garden of Eden. In Christianity, if the fruit is broken or bursting open, it is a symbol of the fullness of Jesus' suffering and resurrection. In Armenia and India, the pomegranate symbolizes prosperity and fertility, and in Hinduism the fruit is associated with both *Bhoomidevi* (the earth goddess) and Lord Ganesha.

In the *Ayurveda*, the pomegranate has been used as a source of traditional remedies for thousands of years. The rind of the fruit and the bark of the pomegranate tree is used as a traditional remedy against diarrhea, dysentery and intestinal parasites. The seeds and juice are considered a tonic for the heart and throat.

Steeped in symbolism since ancient times, it is today heralded as a superfood. Eating a pomegranate with a strong desire in mind is considered a magical act and is sure to grant your wish. [Earth ++]

Pumpkin seeds are one of nature's most perfect foods. They alkalize the body more than any other seed of nut; they boost immunity and help to balance hormones. Native Americans treasured them both for their dietary and medical properties, including their ability to relieve depression through detoxification of the body, as well as prevent various cancers, parasites, and improve numerous bodily functions. [Earth ++]

Quinoa was revered by Incas of South America for centuries. Today, it considered a superfood because of its nutritionally dense profile. Quinoa contains all eight essential amino acids making it a complete source of protein. It is by far the most nutritious of all the "grain-like" and grain foods on the planet and should therefore be a staple in all food yogi diets. [Earth +++]

Rye is one of the Seven Sacred Grains of the ancient world. Although thinner, it is more nutritionally dense than wheat, and because of its strong Earth element it encourages a grounded devotion. [Earth +++]

Saffron is considered the most perfect of all spices. It comes from the stigma of the stunningly beautiful violet crocus flower. During a two-week period in autumn, three stigmas from each flower are handpicked and dried. It takes 225,000 stigmas from 75,000 flowers to produce just a pound of the herb. Eating saffron dispels depression and eliminates psychological inertia, and it was once believed that you could die of "excessive joy" by eating too much of it. Drinking the tea is said to bestow the gift of clairvoyance and greatly enhance the body's healing powers. The alchemists considered saffron the gold of the plant kingdom and believed it carried the "signature" of the great transmuting agent for which the alchemists spent their lives searching. Saffron was sacred to the Egyptian supreme god, Amen, and the Egyptians grew it in their sacred gardens at Luxor. Saffron was also sacred to Eos, the Greek god of the morning light, and the spice has been described as the dawn's light solidified. [Fire +++]

Sage has tremendous primal power and is therefore a powerful guardian of the spirit and healing agent. It was sacred to the Greek gods, Zeus and Jupiter. As a dried herb it is a popular purifier when burned as a smudge stick. When consumed fresh or infused in a tea it inspires artistic expression by stimulating the Throat Chakra. It is an outstanding memory enhancer. Sage helps provide better brain function and has been used in the treatment of cerebrovascular disease for over a thousand years. The herb kills bacteria, aids digestion, reduces high blood sugar, strengthens the nervous system, and is an exceptionally rich source of several B-complex groups of vitamins. [Air +++]

Salt in its purest form is the ultimate spice for grounding, protection, and earthly purification. The best salt to consume is Celtic sea salt or pink Himalayan rock salt. Salt was sacred to the Egyptian gods, Osiris and Set. To the alchemist, salt represents the creative feminine energy, as opposed to the destructive male principle of sulfur.

Regular table salt undergoes a whole lot of processing, wherein it is bleached with toxic solvents, ferrocyanide and aluminum to make it white. This abusive processing ends up stripping the natural salt of important minerals like calcium, potassium, copper, sulfate, iodine, iron, manganese, magnesium, silicon, phosphorus, vanadium and zinc (Mercola). [Earth +++]

Sesame seeds are sacred to the elephant deity Ganesha in Hindu theology and are eaten to increase one's basic life force, which the Hindus believe is the hidden creative energy that accumulates at the bottom of the spine. Sesame seeds are exceptionally rich in calcium, containing more of this "bone food" than whole milk. [Earth ++]

Sunflower was sacred to the Greek deities, Helios, Demeter, and Apollo. It is seen as a blending of heavenly and earthly powers, and is associated with the Crown Chakra. The nutritious seeds carry masculine energy. Juice from the stems of sunflowers is used as an ointment to increase one's morality and integrity. The seeds are alkalizing to the body. [Fire +++]

Turmeric is the root of a plant related to ginger and is revered in India for its antiseptic, blood purifying, anti-oxidant, and anti-inflammatory properties. Because of its distinctive yellow color, it is a common ingredient in sacred Hindu ritual. It is superior as a natural coloring agent and just a pinch can make any curry or cake icing turn yellow. Hawaiian priests have used turmeric in purification rituals for centuries. [Fire ++]

FOOD YOGI SMOOTHIES

The following smoothie recipes were inspired by New York's *Liquiteria* café and will make enough for one or two people. The method for most of them is to blend all the ingredients in a high-powered blender; however, some recipes will require a good juicer. *You can add more water or ice as needed.* The quantities will vary slightly depending on the quality of the fruit or vegetable being used.

The benefits of blending fruits as opposed to juicing is that when blending you get to consume the pulp of the fruit which contains many beneficial nutrients, as well as much needed fiber for cleansing your system. Also, this fiber will help regulate the absorption of sugars into your bloodstream. However, make sure to 'chew' your smoothie before you swallow it, because the chewing action will release saliva and mix important digestive enzymes into the drink.

For those recipes requiring nuts, it is best to place the nuts at base of the blender and then add all other ingredients on top. Monitor the consistency of the smoothie as it blends to see if you need to add more water or "vegan milk".

Do your best to buy organic fruits and vegetables. In some cases, it might be more practical to buy organic frozen fruits, but keep in mind that frozen fruits do not have the Qi energy of fresh fruits. Refer to the "Dirty Dozen" for guidance on what fruits and vegetables are safe to buy conventional.

LIQUID MEALS

NUT MILK
1 cup brazil nuts or almonds[223]

---

[223] Soak nuts overnight and discard water. Remove the skins from the almonds before blending.

3–4 cups of purified water
Pinch of celtic sea salt
¼ tsp. nutmeg powder
¼ tsp. cinnamon
3 Tbsp. agave syrup
1 tsp. sunflower oil
1 banana (optional)
1 vanilla bean (optional)

Method: Blend nuts and water until all nuts are liquefied. Strain the contents through cheesecloth. Keep nut pulp for a cookie recipe. Return "milk" to blender and add all remaining ingredients and blend again. Store in fridge for 4 days. Use this "milk" as the basis for your "vegan milk" smoothies. Alternatives: hemp seeds or oats.

BERRY NICE
1 cup blueberries
1 cup of strawberries
1 banana
1 cup of vegan milk[224]
1 heaped Tbsp. pea protein
1 tsp. flax seed oil
1 cup crushed ice

PEACH FACE
4 peaches
4 strawberries
1 banana
1 tsp. apple cider vinegar (optional) [225]
pinch of cinnamon

---

[224] Organic oat milk and almond milk are best; however, rice milk is a nice light alternative. I do not recommend soy milk. It is best to make your own nut or seed milk. See recipe.

[225] Organic apple cider vinegar. Remember, apples are number one on the "Dirty Dozen" list.

¼ cup aloe vera juice

½ tsp. ginkgo biloba (herb)

1 cup crushed ice

GREEN MONSTER

1 cup blueberries

6 strawberries

2 bananas

1 tsp. apple cider vinegar (optional)

1 Tbsp. green barley powder

1 heaped Tbsp. pea protein

1 Tbsp. activated honey[226] (optional)

1 cup of water

1 cup crushed ice

BLACK BEAUTY

2 bananas

1 cup red grapes (seeded)

1 mango cheek

1 tsp. maca powder

1 Tbsp. molasses

1 cup crushed ice

BULLFIGHTER

2 bananas

1 Tbsp. almond butter

1 cup vegan milk

1 Tbsp. bee pollen (optional)

1 Tbsp. maca powder

1 Tbsp. acai berry concentrate

1 scoop chocolate pea protein

½ cup crushed Ice

MUD WRESTLER

1 cup blueberries

---

[226] The *Manuka* honey from New Zealand is a good choice.

2 bananas
1 cup rice milk
1 tsp. spirulina powder
1 heaped Tbsp. vanilla pea protein
½ cup crushed Ice

PAPPY PARADISE
1 cup papaya
1 peach
1 banana
1 tsp. apple cider vinegar (optional)
½ shredded coconut
1 cup crushed ice
1 tsp. agave syrup or maple syrup (optional)

TROPICAL SNOW
2 oranges (peeled and quartered)
1 banana
1 grapefruit (peeled and quartered)
½ cup aloe vera juice
2 Tbsp. honey or maple syrup
1 Tbsp. colloidal silver[227] (optional)
1 cup water
½ cup ice

COCO BANGO
1 whole baby coconut (water and flesh)
2 bananas
1 small mango
1 Tbsp. pea protein powder
1 tsp. maca powder (optional)
1 tsp. flax seed oil
½ cup ice

---

[227] Colloidal Silver is a liquid suspension of microscopic silver particles and is claimed to be an effective anti viral, anti bacterial agent.

THE HULK SHAKE

This smoothie will power you all day. I take my personal version up a notch by adding some exotic Indian herbs like *Ashwagandha*[228] (virility) and *Brahma Rasayana*[229] (brain food), Saw Palmetto (prostate). Garnish with some goji berries and a mint leaf. This recipe will make enough to fill an entire blender.

> 3 bananas
>
> 1 mango
>
> 2 cup vegan milk (or purified water)
>
> 2 Tbsp. raw almond butter[230] or ½ cup almonds
>
> 3 fresh Kale leaves (remove stems)
>
> 1 Tbsp. maca powder (optional)
>
> 1 tsp. green barley or wheatgrass powder
>
> 1 Tbsp. colloidal silver (optional)
>
> ½ tsp. spirulina powder
>
> ½ tsp. MSM[231] powder (optional)
>
> 2 heaped Tbsp. pea protein powder
>
> ¼ cup raw cacao (nibs[232] or 1 Tbsp. powder)
>
> 2 Tbsp. coconut oil
>
> 1 tsp. flaxseed oil
>
> 4 fresh mint leaves
>
> ½ cup crushed Ice
>
> 1 Tbsp. honey or coconut sugar
>
> 1 tsp. bee pollen (optional)

---

[228] *Withania somnifera*, also known as *Ashwagandha*, Indian ginseng, Winter cherry, Ajagandha, Kanaje Hindi, Amukkara (Tamil), Samm Al Ferakh, is a plant in the Solanaceae or nightshade family. Also known as the "horse herb" and is famed for increasing virility.

[229] *Brahma Rasayan* is a paste consisting of herbs and fruits. It is a cerebral tonic, which strengthens memory and gives energy.

[230] Alternatively, you can use 1 cup of water and ½ cup of fresh raw almonds and ¼ cup of pumpkin seeds.

[231] Methylsulfonylmethane (MSM) is an organosulfur compound with the formula $(CH3)2SO2$. It is also known by several other names including DMSO2, methyl sulfone, and dimethyl sulfone.

[232] Cacao nibs are broken up pieces of cacao seeds.

1 pinch of celtic sea salt

COCO CHAI
1 fresh baby coconut (all the water and "meat")
½ banana
4 medjool dates
2 Tbsp. agave syrup or maple syrup
1 tsp. chai spices
1 tsp. freshly grated ginger
1 cup of crushed ice

FRESH POWER JUICES
You will need a good quality juicer to make some of these super drinks.

BRAIN ZINGER
2 carrots
2 kale leaves
1 red apple
2 cabbage leaves
1 sprig of parsley
1 tsp. ginko

COLD CRUSHER
(hot*/cold)
2 green apples
½ cup grated ginger
1 lemon
1 tsp. ginseng
1 pinch of cayenne (optional)
1 tsp. honey (optional)

GRASSHOPPER
2 apples
1 pear
1 cup of pineapple

1 shot of wheatgrass juice[233]

4 mint leaves

SUMMER BREEZE

2 apples

4 large celery stalks

1 tsp. grated ginger

½ cup ice

GINSENG GO GO

2 carrots

2 apples

2 Tbsp. grated ginger

1 tsp. vitamin C powder

1 tsp. ginseng

1 tsp. bee pollen (optional)

ALIVE AND KICKING

2 carrots

2 large sticks of celery

1 apple

½ beetroot

1 tsp. grated ginger

2 Tbsp. chlorella

THE ROYAL FLUSH

1 cup pineapple

1 pear

2 Tbsp. grated ginger

½ cup aloe vera juice

1 stem of fresh fennel

2 leaves dandelion

1 tsp. MSM powder

1 tsp. colloidal silver

---

[233] Requires Wheatgrass juicer

BEET IT

2 large carrots
½ beetroot
1 apple
1 pear
1 small lemon
1 Tbsp. grated ginger

LIQUID LOZENGER

Use a blender for this recipe. Cut the orange and grapefruit in quarters, peel and place the whole fruit in the blender.

2 Oranges (peeled and quartered)
1 Grapefruit or 2 Lemons
2 Tbsp. grated Ginger
1 Mango cheek
1 stalk of Fennel
1 Tbsp. Honey (optional)
1 cup crushed Ice

REFRESHERS

These are all blender recipes.

MULTIPLE ORANGASM

3 oranges
1 mango
1 cup of strawberries
½ cup aloe vera juice
1 pinch of cayenne
1 pinch of Celtic sea salt
1 Tbsp. honey (optional) or maple syrup
½ cup crushed ice

ARVO D'LITE

1 cup pineapple
1 cup melon
6 mint leaves
1 apple

1 pear

ROOMBA

2 cups mixed berries
1 cup pineapple
1 tsp. apple cider vinegar (optional)
½ cup aloe vera juice
1 tsp. vitamin C powder
1 tsp. maple syrup
1 cup crushed ice

HOLIDAY KISS

1 mango
1 cup strawberries
1 peach
1 tsp. apple cider vinegar (optional)
1 tsp. vitamin C powder
1 pinch cayenne
1 cup crushed ice

LIGHT ENERGY

1 banana
1 cup strawberries
1 tsp. apple cider vinegar
1 heaped Tbsp. pea protein
1 cup crushed ice

POWER PINA COLADA

1 banana
2 cups of pineapple (cubed)
4 strawberries
1 tsp. apple cider vinegar (optional)
1 cup coconut milk[234]

---

[234] Best to make your own using a fresh baby coconut comprising of the coconut water and white coconut "meat" inside the shell which you can scoop out with an ice cream scoop. Otherwise, purchase organic coconut milk or organic coconut water.

It is best to drink these super drinks as soon as possible after making to maximize the nutritional benefits. The important thing to note is that you can fuel your body on a liquid diet. It is a great way to cut calories, and for those of us that live a rushed life, a healthy smoothie in the morning is an efficient way to start the day.

In sharing some smoothie recipes, my hope is that you will begin adding more whole foods into your diet. I am certainly not advocating that you only consume liquid meals. The golden rule is: eat according to your constitution and always seek balance of the five elements (earth, water, fire, air, ether).

For more recipes, including savouries, desserts and breads, go to: facebook.com/foodyogi

Fermented Foods

Fermented and cultured foods are rich in probiotics, enzymes, vitamins and minerals. Plus they're exceptionally easy to prepare. I am including a section on this important food category, because just like freshly made smoothies, eating fermented foods is a very efficient and affordable way of adding easily digestible and concentrated nutrition into your diet.

People have been eating bacteria ridden foods for hundreds of thousands of years. Its part of human history, but modern researchers are just now beginning to understand what the sages of the past knew well: fermented foods offer clear and measurable health benefits to the human diet.

Fermentation (zymology) in food processing is the conversion of carbohydrates to alcohols and carbon dioxide or organic acids using yeasts, bacteria, or a combination thereof, under anaerobic (without oxygen) conditions.

Fermentation usually implies that the action of microorganisms is desirable, and the process has been successfully employed in the leavening of breads; in preservation techniques to produce lactic acid in sour foods such as sauerkraut, kimchi, kombucha and yogurt; and in pickling of foods with vinegar (acetic acid).

French chemist Louis Pasteur was the first known zymologist, when in 1856 he connected yeast to fermentation. Pasteur originally defined fermentation as "respiration without air."

Food fermentation has been said to serve five main purposes:

- Enrichment of the diet through development of a diversity of flavors, aromas, and textures in food substrates
- Preservation of substantial amounts of food through

lactic acid, alcohol, acetic acid, and alkaline fermentations
- Biological enrichment of food substrates with protein, essential amino acids, essential fatty acids, and vitamins
- Elimination of antinutrients
- A decrease in cooking time and fuel requirements

In most agricultural traditions, some form of fermented food is a standard component of the diet. For example, fermented, leavened bread was produced in Ancient Egypt, and milk was fermented in early Babylon as well. Roman soldiers often subsisted on long-fermented sourdough bread, which survived arduous treks in extreme weather.

The list goes on and on: East and Southeast Asia has natto (fermented soy), kimchi (fermented cabbage), soy sauce, to name just a few; Central Asia with kefir (fermented cow milk), and shubat (fermented camel milk); India and the Middle East with fermented pickles, various yogurts, torshi (mixed vegetables); Europe with sauerkraut, and kefir; the Americas with kombucha, standard pickling, and chocolate (fermented cacao); the Pacific region with poi (fermented, mashed taro root) and something called kanga pirau, or rotten corn.

The modern diet is definitely lacking healthful fermented foods and this fact has played a major role in B12 deficiency. James Oswald of *The Institute for Plantbased Nutrition* says, "Healthy individuals recycle B12 in their bodies. Our review of research indicates that it is passed through the digestive tract and then reabsorbed by the colon so that a given supply may last many years. Some colons may not assimilate B12 well and a deficiency might be determined through a blood test. Many so-called nutritional deficiencies are results of assimilation problems rather than effects of insufficient intake."

Don Chisholm, author of *Have you got the guts to be really healthy?* concurs: "We are not what we eat, we are what we absorb and without a good complement of life enhancing bacteria we not only have a compromised system, our digestive system has little chance of extracting the nutrients, vitamins and minerals from food that our cells need."

Oswald explains that all creatures get B12 through inhaling, licking and eating food which has been exposed to air and the particulate matter it carries. "B12 is on, rather than in plants. We sometimes go overboard scouring and peeling, when in fact some of the really good stuff is on the surface of the plant!"

Probiotics

We have a non-human ecosystem within us that is just as, if not more complex than the ecosystem around us.

Our human body is a host to trillions of bacteria, each one of them play a critical role in helping us to function as a living organism. In fact, no living thing on this planet could survive without the help of bacteria. We share a symbiotic relationship with bacteria. Our body's bacteria depend on us to survive and we depend on them to stay alive.

Our digestive system is managed by bacteria, many of which are our first line of defense for our immune system. According to Chisholm, we have over 500 species in our gut alone. The good bacteria that helps build our immunity, does so by protecting our body from unwelcome and harmful bacteria. The more good bacteria we have as opposed to bad bacteria, the less chance we have of getting food poisoning, and the more efficient we are in absorbing the nutrients from food.

Most people today are ignorant about the importance of good bacteria in the body ecosystem. Instead, when disease strikes they load their body ecosystem with pharmaceuticals that mask the problem or antibiotics that indiscriminately destroy all forms of bacteria in the gut, including those that serve as our first line of immune defense.

If you consider that our gut bacteria is what supports our immune system, it becomes obvious that destroying it greatly impacts our ability to fight off disease. Chisholm adds, "A lack of nutrient absorption in our digestive system leads to nutrient-depleted cells, which eventually lead to disease."

One statement by Chisholm particularly caught my eye in this regard. "There should be over 3 ½ pounds (2 kg) of good bacteria in a healthy gut." Aside from antibiotics, there are many other things that kill bacteria, including chlorine, fluoride, pesticides, herbicides, birth control pills, alcohol, and stress.

Simple Sauerkrauts Recipe

Even store bought sauerkrauts are often bastardized through mass production, with the manufacturers using vinegar as a preservative rather than the traditional (and naturally occurring) lacto-bacterial-salt slurry. Many brands are also pasteurized and therefore bereft of the true taste and nutrients typically found in sauerkrauts. It is best to make your own, and the good news is, it is rather easy to make simple sauerkrauts. Here is one recipe.

Ingredients
1 cabbage
1 Tbsp. sea salt (make sure your salt is non-iodized)

Step 1
Remove outer leaves from cabbage and chop or grate with a food processor or box grater.

Step 2
Add shredded cabbage to a large bowl with sea salt. The salt helps pull water out of the cabbage and inhibits any bad bacteria from forming.

Step 3
Knead the cabbage with your hands until the salt is evenly distributed and the cabbage juice begins releasing.

Step 4
Use your fist to pack cabbage with its juices tightly into a wide-mouth canning jar with a metal lid, or a ceramic fermenting crockpot. Press one of the reserved outer leaves into the jar to keep the cabbage submerged in its brine.

Step 5
Cover the jar tightly and allow it to ferment at room temperature for at least 3 days (less if your kitchen is warm, more if cold). Add spices as desired or serve plain.

Store in the refrigerator.

Benefits

Fermented foods introduce helpful probiotics to our guts. There are tons of possible benefits to adding probiotics (whether by supplement or by fermented foods) to your body, including protection from colon cancer, relief from lactose intolerance and rotavirus diarrhea, reduction in children's cavities, and prevention of inflammatory bowel disease. The vitamins (like K2) in kefir for example become more plentiful or more concentrated and more bioavailable. Also, the improved digestion that accompanies a healthier gut means more nutrients, vitamins, and minerals are absorbed, thus allowing even better absorption.

Fermented foods don't introduce anything new to human physiology, they merely address a severe deficit in the modern gut. Therefore, introducing beneficial bacteria into our bodies can restore the balance of intestinal flora that was once upon a time a normal condition for people who ate wholefood diets and exposed themselves to bacteria on a regular basis.

For more information on wild fermented foods, visit: http://www.wildfermentation.com/

CONCLUDING WORDS

The path of the food yogi described in FOOD YOGA is as much about sharing my own personal realizations as it is a call to action for you, the reader, to take this one part of your life – nourishment – and raise it to the highest level. My hope is that by making conscientious food preparation part of your spiritual ritual, and by embracing the culture of spiritual hospitality through sharing *prasadam* with others, you can create the most profound spiritual experiences by nourishing your body, mind and soul, and become a true food yogi.

The founder of Food for Life, Srila Prabhupada, told me that I could literally "eat my way back to Godhead." At first, the statement seemed somewhat absurd, but having imbibed the Vedic culture of spiritual hospitality and then learning of the food rituals of many other great spiritual traditions, I have come to realize that Srila Prabhupada was indeed onto something. Our spiritual awareness does indeed prosper the more we focus on the type of food we eat and how it is prepared, and more importantly, how we control the tongue.

Not only can the art and science of food yoga bring you astounding personal benefits, I believe it has the power to transform an entire world, and realize Srila Prabhupada's vision that through the liberal distribution of *prasadam* and *sankirtan*,[235] "the whole world can become peaceful and prosperous."[236]

---

[235] Sanskrit term, meaning the congregational chanting of the holy names of God.
[236] *Srimad Bhagavatam* Verse 4.12.10 purport.

APPENDIX

- Holy food in the Judeo-Christian tradition
- Offering food in Buddhist tradition
- Mercy and charity in the Islamic tradition
- Eating and charity in the Jewish tradition
- Saint Francis of Assisi
- About the author
- Resources
- Bibliography
- Start your own project

HOLY FOOD IN THE JUDEO-CHRISTIAN TRADITION

By *Chaitanya dasa (Brother Aelred)*

In the Judeo-Christian tradition, as in all other religious traditions, the preparation, offering and consumption of food have a central role. Central is the understanding that God has blessed the earth so that it will be able to produce, and that humanity may be blessed in the eating.

Let us look at a variety of Biblical references to holy food.

There is a vital passage at the end of Chapter 1 of Genesis – the first reference to food in the Bible, and the first reference to the food which has been given to Adam and Eve, our first parents:

> God said, "See, I give you all the seed-bearing plants that are upon the whole earth, and all the trees with seed-bearing fruit; this shall be your food ..."

One Catholic priest said to me recently, "Your commitment to a vegetarian diet is justified by reference to scripture." He was, of course, referring to the above verse. It is very interesting (and disturbing) that Christians consistently overlook (ignore?) this passage, and choose to follow the less desirable diet given following the Great Flood – the diet that allowed meat-eating. Whenever I raise this matter there is an awkward silence ... then a flow of excuses!

In the Old Testament book of Leviticus, Chapter 22, there is a lengthy passage on the subject of holy food:

> Yahweh spoke to Moses; he said: "Speak to Aaron and his sons: let them be consecrated through the holy offerings of the sons of Israel...

> "Any one of your descendants, in any generation, who in a

state of uncleanness approaches the holy offerings consecrated to Yahweh by the sons of Israel, shall be outlawed from my presence...

"...At sunset he will be clean and may then eat holy things, for these are his foods...

"They (lay people) must not profane the holy offerings which the sons of Israel have set aside for Yahweh. To eat these would lay on them a fault demanding a sacrifice of reparation; for it is I, Yahweh, who have sanctified these offerings."

We obviously have a greater interest in the New Testament, especially as it has to do with "the best son of God," Jesus. *Bhagavad-gita* commentator, Srila Prabhupada referred to Jesus in these words. In the New Testament we have two themes of central importance:

1. The sharing of food by believers or devotees. In Acts 2: 42-47 we read the following:

These [the early Christian community] remained faithful to the teaching of the apostles, to the brotherhood, to the breaking of bread and to the prayers.

The faithful all lived together and owned everything in common; they sold their goods and possessions and shared the proceeds among themselves according to what each one needed.

They went as a group to the temple every day but met in their houses for the breaking of bread; they shared their food gladly and generously; they praised God and were looked up to by everyone.

In his First Letter to the Corinthians, St. Paul writes:

Whatever you eat, whatever you drink, whatever you do at all, do it for the glory of God ...

Later in the letter, St. Paul deals at length (chapter 11) with the whole subject of eating food. He is scathing in his criticism of the behavior of   some, specifically because the eating of food is presented in the context of the Eucharist or the Lord's Supper. I will quote the whole passage since, outside the Gospels themselves, it is the most important teaching on the subject of holy food.

The Lord's Supper

> Now that I am on the subject of instructions, I cannot say that you have done well in holding meetings that do you more harm than good. In the first places, I hear that when you all come together as a community, there are separate factions among you, and I half believe it—since there must no doubt be separate groups among you, to distinguish those who are to be trusted. The point is, when you hold meetings, it is not the Lord's Supper that you are eating, since when the time comes to eat, everyone is in such a hurry to start his own supper that one person goes hungry while another is getting drunk. Surely you have homes for eating and drinking in? Surely you have enough respect for the community of God not to make poor people embarrassed? What am I to say to you? Congratulate you? I cannot congratulate you on this.

> For this is what I received from the Lord, and in turn passed on to you: that on the same night that he was betrayed, the Lord Jesus took some bread, and thanked God for it and broke it, and he said, 'This is my body, which is for you; do this as a memorial of me.' In the same way he took the cup after supper, and said, 'This cup is the new covenant in my blood. Whenever you drink it, do this as a memorial of me.' Until the Lord comes, there, every time you eat this bread and drink this cup, you are proclaiming his death, and so anyone who eats the bread or drinks the cup of the Lord unworthily will be behaving unworthily toward the body and blood of the Lord.

> Everyone is to recollect himself before eating this bread and drinking this cup; because a person who eats and drinks without recognizing the Body is eating and drinking his

own condemnation. In fact that is why many of you are weak and ill and some of you have died. If only we recollected ourselves, we should not be punished like that. But when the Lord does punish us like that, it is to correct us and stop us from being condemned with the world.

So to sum up, my dear brothers, when you meet for the Meal, wait for one another. Anyone who is hungry should eat at home, and then your meeting will not bring your condemnation. The other matters I shall adjust when I come.

In conclusion, I would say that *prasadam* holds a central place in the Christian tradition, although with an added dimension. By "added dimension" I mean that, in the Eucharist/Mass/Lord's Supper, not only are bread and wine offered to God, and so set apart from mundane use, they actually manifest the presence of Jesus Christ. Jesus Christ is actually present in every Mass. Indeed the bread and wine are the worshipable form of the Lord. Such is the Catholic and Orthodox doctrine of the "Real Presence."

OFFERING FOOD IN BUDDHIST TRADITIONS

Offering food is an ancient tradition in Buddhism. Monks will often collect food when begging and in order to receive blessings, the public will offer various vegetarian foods before tantric deities.

Offerings Alms to Monks

The early Buddhist monks were homeless mendicants who owned little more than a robe and begging bowl. Today, monks still often rely on receiving alms for most of their food. However, the monks will often not speak, even to say "thank you", and in some sects the monks will cover their faces with large hats so that there is not even eye contact. According to Buddhist doctrine, there is to be no giver and no receiver; just giving and receiving. This purifies the act of giving and receiving, they say. The giving of alms is not thought of as charity, but a means for the public to spiritually connect to the monastic order.

Ceremonial Food Offerings

The rituals and doctrines used in ceremonial food offerings in Buddhism differ widely from one school to another. In the most basic ceremony, food is simply left on an altar, while a more formal offering might involve elaborate chants and full prostrations. However it is done, as with the alms given to monks, the offering is a means of connecting with the spiritual realm. In more practical terms, it is a way to rid the heart of selfishness.

Making food offerings to the hungry ghosts is a common practice in Zen Buddhism. It is said that hungry ghosts represent greed and attachments to this world. By renouncing that which we desire, we release ourselves from the shackles of attachment and neediness.

In the Buddhist *Hinayana* and *Mahayana* traditions, there are three ways of offering food. The *Mahayana* way includes *Vajrayana* or the secret *mantra*. This tradition centers on giving food in charity to all sentient beings, including microbes that live in our bodies.

Lama Zopa Rinpoche, of the *Mahayana* Buddhist tradition explains:

> *Offering food with the motivation "I'm going to practice food yoga and make charity of this food to all sentient beings in order to attain enlightenment for the sake of all sentient beings" is a bodhicitta practice and is based on renunciation of samsara.*

The *Hinayana* tradition of offering food is based on the methods expressed in the prayer by *Nagarjuna*,[237] where he explains that the purpose of eating food is not to grow a strong body from which attachment arises, but rather to survive in order to practice *dharma*.[238] Food, therefore, should be consumed without the three poisonous arrows of ignorance, attachment, and anger. Lama Zopa Rinpoche explains that one's motivation should be to seek freedom from the cycle of reincarnation (*samsara*), by first offering the food to the "Triple Gem"[239] before eating.

Although similar to the Judeo Christian tradition of giving thanks before a meal, the *Hinayana* tradition, like many of the Eastern food traditions, adds a layer of reciprocity to this

---

[237] (ca. 150-250 CE) Indian philosopher who founded the *Madhyamaka* school of Mahāyāna Buddhism.
[238] Sanskrit: One's righteous duty. In modern Indian languages it often means religion. It literally translates as that which upholds or supports, and is therefore often equated with law.
[239] Also called the *Three Treasures* or *Three Refuges*, they are the three things that Buddhists take refuge in, and look toward for guidance. They are: *Buddha, Dharma, Sangha.*

gratitude through a practical expression of giving back to the Creator.

MERCY AND CHARITY IN THE ISLAMIC TRADITION

Whoever is kind to the creatures of God is kind to himself
– Hadith of Prophet Mohammed

Mercy to Animals

Absolutely no killing is allowed as pilgrims approach Mecca, including even lice, ants, grasshoppers and mosquitoes. If a pilgrim sees an insect on the ground, he will gesture his friends to be careful to avoid treading on it. This example illustrates that while Islam is not generally viewed as a religion that promotes vegetarianism and kindness to animals, the Islamic tradition does have a lot to say about how people should relate to the animal world.

Indeed, there are numerous examples of Mohammed showing his compassion to animals. In his *Story of Mohammed the Prophet*, Bilkiz Alladin quotes the Prophet: "Show sympathy to others ... especially to those who are weaker than you." According to other biographical accounts, Mohammed has been quoted as saying, "Where there is an abundance of vegetables, hosts of angels will descend on that place."

Charity

Zakāh (sometimes *Zakāt/Zekat* or "alms giving"), one of the Five Pillars of Islam, is the charitable giving of a small percentage of one's possessions (surplus wealth, including food), generally to poor and needy Muslim individuals. Often compared to the system of tithing and alms, *Zakāh* serves principally as the Islamic welfare service to poor and deprived Muslims, although others are not excluded. The Islamic community has a duty to not only collect *zakat*, but to distribute it equitably as well.

The Quran states:

By no means shall you attain righteousness, unless you give of that which you love[240]

Zakat is sometimes referred to as *sadaqah* and its plural, *sadaqat*. Generally, the sharing of wealth is called *zakat*, whereas *sadqat* can mean sharing wealth or sharing happiness among God's creation, such as speaking kindly, smiling at someone, taking care of animals and the environment, etc.

Zakat or *sadqah* is therefore considered worship and is a means of spiritual purification. It is not seen as a tax burden but rather serves as socio-financial system of Islam by redistributing the wealth among the poor and needy.

There is no disagreement among Muslims about the obligatory nature of *zakat*. It simply must be done. Throughout the Islamic history, denying *Zakat* equals denying the Islamic faith. However, the Muslim jurists differ on many details of *zakat*, each having their own opinion and arguments on matters such as frequency of distribution, exemptions, and the types of wealth that are *zakatable*. Most scholars consider all agricultural products *zakatable*.

Zakat has been compared with such a high sense of righteousness that it is often placed on the same level of importance as offering *Salat*.[241] Muslims also see this act as a way of purifying themselves from greed and selfishness while protecting good business relationships. In addition, *zakat* purifies recipients because it saves them from the humiliation of begging and prevents them from envying the rich. Because *zakat* holds such a high level of importance in the culture, it is

---

[240] Quran 3:92

[241] Ritual prayer (*salat*) which is performed five times each day: at dawn (*al-fajr*), midday (*al-zuhr*), afternoon (*al-'asr*), sunset (*al-maghrib*) and evening (*al-'isha*).

stated, "... the prayers of those who do not pay *zakat* will not be accepted."

There are two categories of charity in Islam: obligatory and voluntary.

Who is entitled to receive zakat

Eight categories of individuals may receive the *zakat*, Noble *Quran* (9:60)

1. The needy (Muslim or non Muslim)- Fuqara'
2. Extremely poor (Muslim or non Muslim—Al-Masakin
3. Those employed to collect – Aamileen
4. Those whose hearts are to be won – Muallafatul Quloob
5. To free the captives—Ar-Riqaab
6. Those in debt (Muslim or non Muslim – Al Ghaarimeen
7. In the way of Allah – Fi Sabeelillah
8. Wayfarers (Muslim or non Muslim) – Ibnus-Sabeel

EATING AND CHARITY IN THE JEWISH TRADITION

The foundational teaching within the Jewish tradition is the Torah's injunction to "eat, be satisfied, and bless YHVH,[242] your God for the good of earth."

It should first be noted how these words honor the very act of eating. In other words, eating is not simply a mundane act of selfishness, an evil necessity, or something we have to do to maintain our bodies; it is holy.

The Talmudic sages taught that the dinner table is like the altar in the temple, and the meal we eat like the offering that brought us close to God.

Jay Michaelson, in *God in Your Body*, explains: "The Hebrew word for such offerings, *korbanot*, comes from the same root as *l'karev*, to be brought close. Rather than "sacrifices," a better translation might be "joiners" or even "unifiers."

"Eating is simple," he continues, but eating in a manner that fulfills the commandment to be satisfied and bless "takes a certain amount of subtraction," or cutting down the noise of an impossible, rushed life.

To eat in this manner requires mindfulness, and the Jewish injunction to meditate while eating endorses this. For example, the *Darchei Tzedek's* statement that "The main service of God is through eating. Moreover the *tzaddikim* (righteous ones) meditate as they eat, in love and fear of God, as with prayer."[243]

---

[242] *Yahweh*

[243] Darchei Tzedik p. 18 Translated by Yitzhak Buxbaum in Jewish Spiritual Practices, p. 226.

The Talmud encourages us to cultivate a moment of sincerity as we consume our food:

The miracle of food that God provides is as spectacular as the splitting of the Red Sea.[244]

"The natural desires of the body are gifts from God," explains Michaelson. He quotes the Hasidic master Rabbi Zusya of Hanipol, who said:

The will of the Creator, blessed be He then, is to "enliven every thing" for I am doing His will by eating ... It is God who has brought you to this hunger and thirst. For the hunger is from God.[245]

Finally, medieval Jewish sage Bahya ibn Pakuda, from his masterpiece, *The Duties of the Heart*, writes:

Whoever contemplates the natural processes of the body – how when food enters it, it is distributed to every part of the body – will see such signs of wisdom that he will be inspired to thank the Creator and praise Him, as David said,

All of my bones shall say: "God, who is like You!" (Psalms 35:10)

He will see how food passes into the stomach through a straight tube, called the esophagus, without any bend or twist; how afterwards the stomach digests the food more thoroughly than chewing had; how then the food is carried through thin connecting veins that act as a strainer, preventing anything course from passing through to the liver; how the liver converts the food it receives into blood, which is distributes all over the body through tubes that look like water pipes and were formed specifically for this

---

[244] *Pesachim* 118a.
[245] Quoted in *Mazkeret Shem HaGedolim* (M. H. Kleinman, ed.), p. 79 Translated by Buxbaum in *Jewish Spiritual Practices*, p 231.

purpose ... Meditate, my brother, on the Creator's wisdom in structuring your body.[246]

Giving Charity (Tzedakah)

Judaism places great stress on the giving of charity. The Hebrew word for charity (*tzedakah*) literally means justice. In the Jewish tradition, *tzedakah* is the fulfillment of a commandment to respect a fellow human being as having equal status before God. The Torah states, "Love thy neighbor as thyself" (Lev.19:18), however, the Jewish tradition recognizes that the sharing of resources is more than an act of love, but also an act of justice. This is to emphasize the point that the needy are entitled to our love and compassion, because they too are created in the image of God and have a purpose within God's creation.

---

[246] Rabbi Bahya ibn Pakuda, *The Duties of the Heart*, Gate of Discernment, Chapter 5, translated into Hebrew by R. Yehuda ibn Tibbon in Haberman, ed., p. 196.

SAINT FRANCIS OF ASSISI

There are basically two distinct schools of Christian thought: The *Aristotelian-Thomistic* school and the *Augustinian-Franciscan* school.

The *Aristotelian-Thomistic* school teaches that animals are here for our pleasure—they have no independent purpose. We can eat them; torture them in laboratories – whatever we feel is necessary for our survival. Most modern Christians embrace this form of their religion.

The *Augustinian-Franciscan* school, however, teaches that all living beings are brothers and sisters under God's fatherhood. Based largely on the teachings of St. Francis, this platonic worldview fits neatly within the vegetarian perspective.

St. Francis felt a deep kinship with all of creation, addressing it as a "brother" or "sister," firmly believing that everything came from the same creative Source.

His great compassion and respect for the animal world also manifest in his expression of hospitality during Christmas (1223):

> And on Christmas Eve, out of reverence for the Son of God, whom on that night the Virgin Mary placed in a manger between the ox and the ass, anyone having an ox or an ass is to feed it a generous portion of choice fodder. And, on Christmas Day, the rich are to give the poor the finest food in abundance.

Indeed, St. Francis' respect for creation appeared to have no boundaries. It is said that he once removed worms from a busy road and placed them to the side so they would not be crushed under human traffic.

When mice ran over his table as he took his meals or over his body while he slept, he regarded the disturbance as a "diabolical temptation" which he met with patience and restraint, indicating his compassion towards other living creatures.

The Catholic Encyclopedia comments on his compassion:

St. Francis' gift of sympathy seems to have been wider even than St. Paul's, for we find no evidence in the great Apostle of a love for nature or for animals ... Francis' love of creatures was not simply the offspring of a soft sentimental disposition. It arose from that deep and abiding sense of the presence of God. To him all are from one Father and all are real kin ... hence, his deep sense of personal responsibility towards fellow creatures: the loving friend of all God's creatures.

According to St. Francis, a lack of compassion for animals leads to a lack of mercy towards humans. "If you have men who will exclude any of God's creatures from the shelter of compassion and pity, you will have men who will deal likewise with their fellow men," he said.

These wise words ring true in a modern world that kills tens of billions of animals annually. It appears that a nonchalant attitude towards animals could indeed be the root cause of an indifference to the fact that nearly one billion humans go hungry every day.

The Reverend Basil Wrighton, who served as Chairman of the Catholic Study Circle for Animal Welfare in London, during the 1960s, called St. Francis *"the greatest gentleman that Christianity has produced, in the strictest sense of the word."* Reverend Wrighton himself was a remarkable figure, writing in favor of vegetarianism, against animal experimentation, decades before the contemporary movement for animal rights emerged.

According to the Reverend Alvin Hart, an Episcopal priest in New York:

Many Georgian saints were distinguished by their love for animals. St. John Zedazneli made friends with bears near his hermitage; St. Shio befriended a wolf; St. David of

Garesja protected deer and birds from hunters, proclaiming, 'He whom I believe in and worship looks after and feeds all these creatures, to whom He has given birth.' Early Celtic saints, too, favored compassion for animals. Saints Wales, Cornwall and Brittany of Ireland in the 5th and 6th centuries AD went to great pains for their animal friends, healing them and praying for them as well.

One of the many anomalies of so-called civilized society is the convenient justification of some people to eat certain socially-acceptable forms of meat while simultaneously working to protect animals. Otoman Zar-Adusht Ha'nish,[247] said it this way:

It is strange to hear people talk of humanitarianism, who are members of societies for the prevention of cruelty to children and animals, and who claim to be God-loving men and women, but who, nevertheless, encourage by their patronage the killing of animals merely to gratify the cravings of appetite.

---

[247] Otoman Zar-Adusht Ha'nish (1844–1936) was the founder of the religious health movement known as *Mazdaznan*, which is based on Zoroastrian and Christian ideas with special focus on breathing exercises, vegetarian diet and body culture.

ABOUT THE AUTHOR

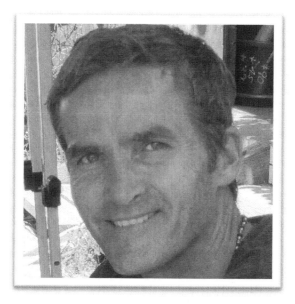

Paul Rodney Turner (the Food Yogi) is the international director of Food for Life and the founder of Food for Life Global, the world headquarters for the charity.

Paul was born in Sydney, Australia in 1963 and grew up in Whalan, a housing commission area of Sydney's Western Suburbs.

As a young boy, Paul enjoyed seeing his father Rod Turner make food for his friends. Rod was a colorful character and never missed an opportunity to pull a prank on his friends. Without fail, when a friend came to visit, Paul's father would offer them something to eat. However, his gesture of hospitality always had a devious agenda. The snack was usually a toasted sandwich consisting of leftover curry or pasta, but laced with the hottest chilies he could find! "My dad was a typical Australian larrikin.[248] Seeing grown men cry while enjoying every bite was pretty funny."

---

[248] A person given to comical or outlandish behavior.

At the age of 19, Paul left home to live in an artists' commune called *Art Haven* in Sydney's famous Blue Mountains. Some local artists had taken over an abandoned holiday resort in Blackheath and had sent word out for other artists to come and join them. Looking for any excuse to get away from the abrasive life he had come to expect in Mount Druitt, Paul, his older brother, Daniel and best friend, Jeff Cassels took up the offer. During his time at *Art Haven*, Paul met Akrura das, a former Hare Krishna monk who used to cook at the Krishna temple in Sydney. Akrura introduced Paul to the fundamentals of Indian cooking, and it was this experience that fueled Paul's desire to one day become a temple chef.

Soon after, Paul took a vow of celibacy, joining the Krishna ashram in Colo River, rural New South Wales. For the next 14 years, Paul, now known as *Priyavrata das* by his fellow Vaisnava monks, studied the ancient teachings of the *Vedas* as taught by His Divine Grace A.C. Bhaktivedanta Srila Prabhupada.

In the early years of Paul's life as a monk, he learned gourmet vegetarian cooking under the stewardship of fellow monk Garuda and assisted at the free vegetarian café in Parramatta known as *Gopals*. A few years later, he was cooking the Sunday feasts for the Sydney Hare Krishna temple, sometimes for as many as 300 guests. His desire to focus exclusively on India's Vedic culture of hospitality inspired him to start his own outreach project. At the time, Food for Life was a fledgling food relief organization with programs in Australia, USA, Western Europe and India.

In 1986, Paul started a Food for Life club at the Sydney University where he and other monks provided a hot lunch to hundreds of students three times a week. "The purpose of the club was to give the students a taste for higher vibrational food and to encourage them to change their diet."

In 1989, his food yogi journey took him to Sydney's Hunter Valley region. There he started a new Food for Life program that also included employing chronically unemployable youth to grow organic vegetables for the local Food for Life project, to which the New South Wales State Government awarded a grant of AU$120,000.

Through Paul's efforts to raise funds and awareness of Food for Life during that time, he began to see how food was a wonderful communicator. "Whenever I met anyone I would always have snacks to share, and soon it became so synonymous that the sight of me would bring a smile to people's faces."

Paul's enthusiasm to promote the work of the charity led to appearances on Australia's famous *Ray Martin Show*, numerous radio and other television interviews and a guest appearance on celebrity Andrew Denton's show, *Money or the Gun*.

In 1991, Paul organized a parade and picnic in Kings Cross, Sydney, to celebrate the serving of the 2 millionth free meal by Hare Krishna Food for Life. The guests of honor included the Mayor of Sydney, Vic Smith; Chief inspector of Police, Jim McClosky; and local Member of Parliament Ms. Clover Moore.

It was these firsthand experiences that convinced Paul of food's power to unite and create peace in the world. He later adopted this philosophy when establishing the international headquarters for the charity in Washington DC in 1995. Food for Life Global's slogan became "*Uniting the World Through Pure Food*". The message perfectly captured the soul of Food for Life and the Vedic culture of spiritual hospitality that is founded on the principle of the spiritual equality of all beings.

Over the next 25 years, Paul travelled to more than 50 countries throughout Europe, Asia, and the Americas, helping to inspire and set up new Food for Life projects and train volunteers. He also raised millions of dollars in funds; gave hundreds of public lectures; appeared on television and radio, and met with numerous government officials. In 1994,

Paul wrote the official Food for Life training manual and, in 1996, he wrote, sung and produced the first official FFL music CD called *Prasada Sevaya* (Service to holy food).

From 1999 to 2003, Paul was a Council Member and Magazine Editor for IVU (International Vegetarian Union), the official umbrella organization for vegetarianism worldwide.

During Paul's travels he also visited three war zones: Chechnya, Sarajevo and Sukhumi. In 2005, Paul led an international team of volunteers to set up makeshift kitchens in villages across Sri Lanka in response to the Asian tsunami, where volunteers served freshly cooked vegan meals to tens of thousands.

In 2010, Paul directed an international relief effort in Haiti, where Food for Life Global served thousands of organic vegan meals to hungry Haitians.

Later that same year, Paul published an instructional book for volunteers wishing to start their own Food for Life project, called *How to Build a Great Food Relief*. In the following year he released a new edition of the Food for Life training manual.

Now some 30 years later, Paul continues to serve the expansion of Food for Life projects around the world as a volunteer. His most recent adventure was to establish a feeding program in Japan for the survivors of the 2011 tsunami.

Blog: www.paulrodneyturner.com
Official Book site: www.foodyogi.org
Charity Web site: www.FFL.org
Numerology site: www.soulyantra.com
Billiards site: www.billiardaimtrainer.com

RESOURCES

- Food for Life Global: www.ffl.org
- Food Yoga: www.foodyogi.org
- Organic Consumers Association: www.organicconsumers.org
- Institute for Responsible Technology: www.seedsofdeception.com
- Working Villages International: www.workingvillages.org
- Natural Solutions Foundations: www.healthfreedomusa.org
- List of Vegan certified companies: www.vegan.org
- Veganic Gardening: www.gentleworld.org
- CSA Directory: www.localharvest.org
- Vedas Online: www.vedabase.net
- Conscious Consumers' Network: www.consciousconsumers.net

BIBLIOGRAPHY

- *Bhagavad-gita As It Is*, A.C. Bhaktivedanta Swami Prabhupada. Original Edition, published by Macmillan 1972
- *Inner Paths to Outer Freedom*, Rick Strassman, Slawek Wojtowicz, Luis Eduardo Luna, and Ede Frecska
- *Shamanic Mysteries of Egypt*, Nicki Skully and Linda Star Wolf
- *The Path of the Dream Healer*, ADAM
- *Mysticism and the New Physics*, Michael Talbot
- *The Holographic Universe*, Michael Talbot
- *CUSCO, the Gateway to Inner Wisdom*, Dianne Dunn
- *The Psychic Energy Codex*, Michelle Belanger
- *Diet for Transcendence*, Steven Rosen
- *Holy Cow*, Steven Rosen
- *God in Your Body*, Jay Michaelson
- *In Defense of Food*, Michael Pollan
- *The Alchemical Properties of Food*, Dennis William Hauck
- *Savor, Mindful Eating, Mindful Life*, Thich Nhat Hanh and Lilian Cheung
- *Creative Visualization*, Shakti Gawain
- *The Earth Was Flat*, Mason Howe Dwinell
- *Water – The Ultimate Cure*, Steve Meyerowitz
- *Gluttony*, Francine Prose
- *Raw Food for Real People*, Rod Rotondi
- *Pulse and Water – The Quest*, Don Tolman
- *Sacred Sounds*, Ted Andrews
- *The Top 100 Healing Foods*, Paul Bartimeus
- *The Yoga of Offering Food*, Lama Zopa Rinpoche
- *Food for the Soul: Vegetarianism and the Yoga Traditions*, Steven Rosen
- *Yoga and Vegetarianism: The Path to Greater Health and Happiness*, Sharon Gannon and Ingrid Newkirk
- *Bhagavat Purana*, A.C. Bhaktivedanta Swami Prabhupada. BBT
- *The Higher Taste*, BBT
- *Biblical Vegetarianism*, Vasu Murti Das
- *Love the Animals*, Reverend Andrew Linzey
- *Have you got the guts to be really healthy?* Don Chisolm
- *Earthling, VERITAS (Sept/Oct Issue)*, Martin Zucker
- *PROOF of HEAVEN, A Neurosurgeon's Journey into the Afterlife*, Eben Alexander M.D.

- *Naked Chocolate*, David Wolfe and Shazzie
- *The Astral Plane (Theosophical Manuals)*, Charles W. Leadbeater
- *King James Bible*
- *Mahanirvana Tantra*
- *Qur'an*
- *Sutta Nipata*